final moments

final moments

Nurses' Stories about Death and Dying

Deborah Witt Sherman, PhD, APRN, ANP, BC, ACHPN, FAAN
Editor

KAPLAN) PUBLISHING

© 2009 Kaplan, Inc.

Published by Kaplan Publishing, a division of Kaplan, Inc.
1 Liberty Plaza, 24th Floor
New York, NY 10006

Printed in the United States

Library of Congress Cataloging-in-Publication Data

Final moments : nurses' stories about death and dying /
[edited by] Debora Witt Sherman.
        p. ;   cm. -- (Kaplan voices)
    ISBN 978-1-4277-9823-7
1. Terminal care. 2. Nursing. I. Sherman, Deborah Witt. II. Series.
[DNLM: 1. Attitude to Death--Personal Narratives. 2. Nursing Care--
psychology--Personal Narratives. 3. Nurse-Patient Relations--Personal
Narratives. 4. Terminal Care--psychology--Personal Narratives.
WY 152 F4905 2009]
    RT87.T45F56 2009
    155.9'37--dc22

                                                    2008041278

10 9 8 7 6 5 4 3 2 1

ISBN-13: 978-1-4277-9823-7

Kaplan Publishing books are available at special quantity discounts to use for sales promotions, employee premiums, or educational purposes. Please email our Special Sales Department to order or for more information at kaplanpublishing@kaplan.com, or write to Kaplan Publishing, 1 Liberty Plaza, 24th Floor, New York, NY 10006.

Contents

Introduction

In *Final Moments*, nurses reveal "glimpses behind the curtain," as they bear witness to the final days of their patients' lives, learn to appreciate the sanctity of life, and discover how to face death with dignity. Nurses understand that dying and death may be an opportunity for growth, self-actualization, and healing.

Final Moments is a collection of powerful stories that reveals the lived experiences of nurses from all over the country, in various clinical settings as they care for seriously ill and dying patients. The stories are snapshots that capture the intense emotional and spiritual connection of nurses, patients, and families.

For many, the desire to become a nurse began in early childhood when she or he witnessed the death of a beloved family member. From that point forward, having coped with their own loss and grief, they were "called" to accompany individuals through the illness experience, with a need to celebrate life while preparing for death. In the story entitled "Never Too Late," Rachel Shinabarger tells us about the experiences of student nurses and how they are expected to provide physical, emotional, and spiritual care to dying patients, yet are unprepared educationally or emotionally for the experience. Other nurses seek experiences in the care of the dying as their hearts rejoice when they can alleviate suffering and provide true presence to patients and families.

Nurses' own personal issues of loss and grief create the emotional space to understand the needs, fears, hopes, and dreams of patients and families as they face death. In the story, "There Are No Coincidences," Patrice Piretti describes how nurses identify with patients close to their own age or who share a common heritage. She explains how nurses memories of beloved family members are often awakened by patients who shared similar characteristics and represent the spirit of their heritage. In the story, "Changing Seasons," Terry Ratner describes the need for connection with a patient: the relationship "soothed her broken heart." In this story, we learn that nurses may perceive death as either "coming too soon," or as "freedom from pain."

In the story entitled "She Inspired Me," we understand that nurses are "angels" but that patients are "angels," too. The relationship between a nurse and patient is reciprocal as both hearts are joined in faith and hope to create opportunities for healing.

Openness and trust endear patients and nurses to one another. When nurses encourage patients and families to tell their own life story, nurses demonstrate their respect for the patient's unique life and provide validation for their life experience. Mary DeLisle-Berry, in the story "He's

Coming," describes how nurses gain insight into family dynamics and long standing family conflicts. With such knowledge, nurses can facilitate communication, which may move families to resolve disagreements or at least call a truce for the good of the dying person. As role models, many nurses reveal ways of supporting families at a time when they need to also support each other.

In the story entitled "House Call," Cortney Davis tells us how families rely on the clinical judgment of nurses and await their assessments anticipating the unimaginable—and are gently prepared by nurses as to what to expect. Patients and families ask nurses, "What would you do in this situation?" As revealed in these stories, nurses individualize their approach to care, helping patients and families to understand their own choices based on their personal wishes and preferences, while recognizing the burden and benefits related to each treatment decision. Nurses realize that the voices of patients must be heard, and at times nurses become the voices of patients as they advocate for their best interest within the health care system.

Many of the stories, including "Mel's Story," written by Pato Cog, tell us that nurses are "receivers" as well as "givers" in the care of dying patients and families. Nurses learn from patients how to die with dignity—maintaining a positive attitude despite physical and emotional suffering and how life and its joys should never be taken for granted. Patients teach nurses about "living in the moment" and the importance of not burying them, until they are dead. Many of the nurses in these stories understand that people can actualize their potential even as death approaches— leaving a legacy for families and imprinting the hearts of nurses.

Several of the stories show us how nurses suffer when their patients suffer—never forgetting what they have witnessed. This is found in "Wicked Codes" by Karen Klein and in Emily McGee's "An End to the Madness," as nurses witness painful procedures that are attempted over and over again.

Yet, nurses find their voices in protection of their patients, advocating for an end to painful treatments, while offering comfort and reassurance when the procedure is requested by the patient or deemed necessary by the medical staff. As described in the story entitled "Pearls," Sarah Burns reveals that nurses often wish that they had their "own magic wand" to alleviate pain caused by the disease itself or its treatment. The magic wand of nurses becomes a wand that offers hope, not for cure, but for connection, and opportunities for healing on emotional, social, and spiritual levels.

In bearing witness to suffering, nurses often struggle with their own post-traumatic stress. Davis, who also wrote the "First Night" reveals the fear and anxieties of nurses who are frightened by their own inexperience in caring for seriously ill patients, often questioning their own abilities and fearing that they have contributed to the patient's death. They ask, "What could I have done differently" or "How could I have saved him?" This line of questioning is evident when an expert nurse, as described by Adrienne Zurub in the story "Tender Mercy" badgers herself and laments that she was unable to save her own mother. As readers, we come to understand that personal and professional experiences of loss and grief are closely connected. We learn that death experiences not only can overwhelm novice or student nurses, but those with years of experience. In Zurub's story, we also learn how other health professionals may be unaware of another's emotional pain and that it is the rituals of the operating room which create a mask for grief following the death of the author's mother.

Anne Webster, in her story "The First Patient," tells us that death may be viewed as a failure of nurses' abilities to protect the patient—and in such situations the nurse reveals feelings of remorse and guilt at being unable to do more to save a patient. We learn of the nurse's desire for greater knowledge, and the further development of their clinical skills. But Webster explains that nurses need to learn that death is not a failure, but that nurses simply do the best they can for patients and that life and death are not always in their control. In her story "God Bless the Child," Cara Muhlhahn reminds us, once again, that death may be unavoidable no matter how skilled are the nurses and other members of the health care team, nor the availability of medical technology. Babies and children do die and that death may be unexpected. In telling her story about "Carol," Geraldine Gorman recognizes that people die in the prime of their lives and that life must be celebrated every day. A critically important message is expressed in a story written by Linda L. Lindeke, called "Susie's Story" as the author reminds us that the nurses' role is to listen, offer support, serve as an advocate and help patients negotiate the health care system.

The most important role of the nurse is to "Just Be There"—be present to the patient and to their family in their most difficult hours. Yet, care of the dying patient is not without its pain for the nurse. In "Caring for Mr. B," Nkiru Onyenwe Okammor tells us that nurses may feel confident caring for dying patients, but have difficulty in caring for a deceased person and thereby need the support of their nurse colleagues. Keith Carlson in his story "A Nurse's Recovery from Grief" explains how nurses bring to their practice their own personal experiences of loss and grief and that grieving is a process with physical, emotional, psychological, and spiritual manifestations. He suggests that the "tool kit" to cope with grief includes writing/journaling, psychotherapy, mindfulness mediation, exercise, and short-circuiting negative thoughts that bring distress. This story emphasizes that nurses must continue to care for themselves in ways that honor their grief and trust their inner sense of "right action."

Susan Riker Dolan and Audrey Riker Vizzard tell us "It Doesn't Have to Hurt" either for the patient or the nursing staff. They remind us that palliative and hospice care offers physical, emotional, social and spiritual support of both patient and family and that nurses and other team members are supported by each other as they face loss and grief issues. Shinabarger emphasizes that as nurses "we must allow our own tears," while Carlson reminds us that "grief is a process that is elongated, tangential, and circuitous" and that it is riddled with potholes and bumps that challenge a nurses's recovery.

Yet, nurses' grief often makes them more sensitive to the losses and grief of others—capable of providing healing care which involves a "sense of vibrant energy, use of humor and laughter to raise the spirits, and which provides patients and families encouragement and comfort in living life and facing death with dignity. In the story entitled "Defining Moments," Lisa Affatato speaks of the heart connection between a nurse and patient as nurses are willing to speak about life and death and to offer comfort through touch and words of encouragement and support. In "Whistles over the Rainbow," Patricia Coates Kavanaugh portrays dying as a sacred time in which we learn about life and about each other. Dying patients often share with nurses the peace they experience as they feel the presence of those who have already "crossed over" to an afterlife and who have come to "push them over the rainbow." As death approaches, patients may become too weak and frail to communicate with words but their eyes speak of their love and appreciation for a nurses' gentle care.

These special stories reveal the strong connection between nurses and their patients and highlight the importance of the patient in the lives of nurses, as "patients contribute rich threads to the personal tapestry of nurses' lives." One of the most important lessons learned through this collection of nurse's stories, is that the level of caring between the patient and nurse can influence their individual journey and demonstrate respect for each others' human spirit. This mutual respect creates an environment of trust that strengthens the bonds and contributes to the healing process for both the patient and the nurse. Each story provides "a glimpse behind the curtain," to understand not only the inner life of patients as they face death, but the ways that nurses cope with the loss and death of patients. Although "nurses' hearts may be broken," they continue to love and open their hearts to new patients and, once again we see that the love connection is everlasting, as love has great power in life and in death.

Final Moments

As My Aunt, the Nurse, Lay Dying

∼

Madeleine Mysko, RN

My ELDERLY AUNT lay dying in St. Joseph Hospital, where she was receiving consistently kind and appropriate care from the staff.

Another way to begin the story: My elderly aunt—a registered nurse herself, trained by the Sisters of St. Francis during the 1940s at "the old St. Joseph's" downtown (which had years ago been torn down)—lay dying in a hospital bed just a few miles from home. Her home had been a narrow row house with no bathroom on the first floor, a home from which her family had recently been trying to pry her, because it didn't make sense anymore for her to be living there alone. But those troubles were all behind us now, because my aunt was dying.

From the beginning, then, the story gets complicated, as all personal stories do. It is told from the point of view of the *nurse*—for I am a nurse too, a 1967 graduate of a Catholic hospital nursing school. It is told also from the point of view of the *niece*, the one who sat at the bedside in the hospital room those final days and nights, the one who had to come to terms with the dying of the beloved aunt.

Another way to begin this story, since it is as much about me as it is about my aunt: As a child I was deeply affected by reading *Cherry Ames, Student Nurse,* which was first published in 1943, three years before I was born. Or rather, I should say, I was deeply affected by a certain passage either in *Cherry Ames, Student Nurse,* or in another book from the Cherry Ames series, for I admit that in all these years I've never gone back to verify that this passage exists as I remember it. For all I know, the passage doesn't exist at all. It could very well be a product of my childhood imagination, a crucial insight I didn't know enough to write down, but instead pressed between the pages of memory in *Cherry Ames, Student Nurse.*

Before I go further, I should point out that contemporary students of Cherry Ames—feminists and nursing educators in particular—have championed her spunky character and her independent approach to assignments in places as diverse as a U.S. Army post, a dude ranch, and a ski resort. I point this out now because the Cherry Ames passage I remember best isn't about a spunky nurse striding into a fast-paced plot.

No, the passage I've carried in memory all these years is just a simple description of a hospital ward, and of the simple tasks assigned to Miss Cherry Ames. It's a passage that nurses of my aunt's generation would find affirming, and that nurses of my own generation would find on the one hand nostalgic, reminiscent as it is of the old hospitals we were trained in, and on the other hand quaint—amusing even—given the significant changes in our professional lives since 1968, when the last book in the Cherry Ames series was written.

In the passage I remember, it is early morning. Miss Ames walks down the hall of the hospital ward dressed in her starched apron and cap, her polished white shoes squeaking against the shining linoleum. She is carrying fresh linens, perfectly folded and regimentally stacked—a white cord bedspread, two flat sheets, one draw sheet, a pillowcase, a bath blanket, a bath towel, a washcloth, and a bureau scarf.

It is the bureau scarf I remember best, and how after Miss Ames had so cheerfully bathed her patient and made up the bed, she then wiped the patient's little bureau with a damp cloth, and finally laid down the crisp white bureau scarf, on which to set the clean water glass and pitcher clinking with ice.

To return now to where I began: My elderly aunt lay dying—comatose—in St. Joseph Hospital, where she was receiving consistently kind and appropriate care from the staff. I was keeping vigil at the bedside. Sometimes I sat in the company of my aunt's children, my cousins.

Sometimes I sat alone. In the end—when the dying had dragged out a good deal longer than any of us had imagined it would—we'd split the vigil into shifts, so that none of us went without sleep.

I was not afraid of my aunt's approaching death. As a nurse, I knew what to expect, and could see that the staff had made every effort to see to her comforts. Moreover, as a devoted niece, I was hoping that soon my aunt would give up the long struggle and slip into peace. She was a person of deep Catholic faith. It wasn't a stretch to picture her happily entering the communion of saints, somewhere beyond the changing skies that her hospital window framed.

And yet I was not a happy keeper of the bedside vigil. I had no real work to occupy my hands or my mind, and so I was vulnerable there—just looking around and thinking too much. The weight of my aunt's dying bore down on me then. I began to mourn something I couldn't really name, except to say that it was missing from the room where my aunt was taking her slow and shallow breaths, her final breaths.

One morning, while I sat there alone, a new nurse came in. She was young and pretty. She was wearing a snap-front jacket in a fabric my aunt would have liked, tastefully patterned as it was with bouquets of roses and daisies.

The nurse was friendly in a professional sort of way. She wore a name tag that identified her as "R.N." and declared her first name was "Kay."

Kay made a quick assessment of my aunt's condition. She took her blood pressure, checked the oxygen flow, and adjusted the tubing so that it sat perfectly level on my aunt's dusky lip.

"Are you her daughter?" she asked, turning to me with her head slightly tilted, her lips pressed into a half-smile of pity.

"No," I said, "her niece."

And then I said what I said to everyone who came into the room—the one who drew the blood, the one who mopped the floor around the bed, the one who came with the Holy Communion wafer that my aunt was too far gone to take into her mouth. "She's a nurse, you know," I said, "a St. Joe's nurse. She trained at the old hospital, down on Caroline Street."

Kay smiled, but I could see that Caroline Street meant nothing to her. She was probably unaware there had ever been an "old St. Joe's." I could tell she was a good nurse, though, the sort who care enough to pay attention and muster up some sense of the person my aunt had been, before old age and infirmity had put an end to all that.

"I'm a nurse too," I said, making sure to soften the tone of it, so Kay wouldn't worry I'd be the pain in the neck that some family-members-who-also-happen-to-be-nurses can be.

Kay only smiled. She put a hand on my aunt's head, on the wispy white hair that barely covered her scalp. My aunt's hair had always been thin. Long ago she'd parted it in middle, and brushed it into a bun at the nape of her neck. When she dressed for work at the hospital—in a long-sleeved white uniform with cuff links and a collar that got sent separately to the cleaners for extra starch—she would set the stiff organdy ruffles of her nurse's cap exactly halfway up the part, and anchor the arrangement cleanly with a small pearl hat pin.

"I'm sure it's hard," Kay said then, before she had to go.

"Yes," I said. "Thank you."

The only way to end the story: With the image. What I missed—what I mourned the loss of in the room where my aunt lay dying—was the stack of fresh linens, carried in the arms of a nurse, piled against the bib of her crisp white apron. What I missed most of all was the pristine bureau scarf, which would have been ironed in the laundry room down in the hospital basement, somewhere beyond the morgue, beyond the squeak of white shoes, which I can hear even now as I write—white shoes going down the polished floors of a certain kind of ward, the kind my aunt knew long ago, in the old St. Joe's on Caroline Street.

House Call

~

Cortney Davis, MA, RN-C, APRN

Even from my position at the doorway I could see that he was clearly lifeless, a blank look replacing his usual grimace. His wife had been calling the office all afternoon, every half hour, then every 15 minutes. The last call had been one of sheer panic. "I can't wake him up," she said. "I think maybe this is it. Please. Please come right away."

A nurse practitioner, I'd been making house calls to Mr. Cardone for months, examining him at home when he was unable to come to our office. I'd seen him through his surgery, his radiation, and then the last-ditch chemo that didn't cure him but only made him melt, it seemed, into himself. Every week, I'd watched him become a smaller, frailer version of himself.

Now, his wife's anxious voice, her *I think maybe this is it,* told me that he was most certainly dying. I knew that Mrs. Cardone, although expecting this moment—almost wishing for this moment—was not, now that the moment had arrived, sure she could endure it. And so I rushed through my last patient visit of the day and quickly drove the winding back roads to the Cardones' brick house on the lake. The late May day was lovely—the trees still in their new-spring green—and I couldn't help thinking that it was, perhaps, a good day to die: better than a cold, iced-in day in January; better than a rain-soaked, windy day in April. When I pulled into their driveway, I saw Mrs. Cardone appear briefly at the window, waving me in. In a moment, I was standing at the open screen door.

Martin—"Manny" to his friends and family—was lying on the couch, face up, arms folded over his chest as if he were napping. He was dressed in fleece pajamas, too heavy for this warm day but the only clothes that could keep him from shivering, could keep his thin legs and veiny arms from trembling. He had one slipper on; the other had fallen to the floor.

Mrs. Cardone now stood in the far corner of the living room, looking not at him but at me; beside her, almost hidden behind her skirts, stood their grand-daughter, Rebecca. Even during these days of illness, this time of distress, Manny and his wife continued to care for six-year-old Rebecca while their daughter worked. What, I wondered, had Rebecca seen and heard, living so close to her dying grandfather? Like her grandmother,

Rebecca looked not at Manny but at me. Both of them seemed afraid to move closer to him, afraid even to cry for him—knowing, and yet not really knowing, that he was gone. Somehow, I was needed to make this official: a verified death; the end of a 49-year marriage and the end of a long and cumbersome illness.

This wasn't the first time I'd gone to someone's home, making the house call that made official what the family suspected. Every time had been different and yet, in some ways, every time had been the same. I'd learned how to go slowly through the motions of checking the pupils, hollow and staring; of listening for heart sounds and hearing only their strange absence; of auscultating lungs that did not rise and fall, automatically, as they had for a lifetime. As I leaned over Manny I could hear, in the background, the sounds of a washing machine, the hum transmitted through his chest to my ears. Perhaps Mrs. Cardone, eager to maintain some sort of routine, unable to stop to contemplate the lack of momentum that is death, had done some laundry. Perhaps she asked Rebecca, as a distraction, to help her.

I'd also learned, in all the times I'd bent, silent, over the dead, that there are few words necessary to confirm the fact that death has actually occurred. It takes only a look up at the family, a brief *I'm sorry*. These words always draw the family in, closer to the bodies of their loved ones, as if, before, there had been something fearful there, something not quite alive and yet not certainly dead. Somehow, those two words allow the family to move past fear, past that awful suspension of time, into the here and now. Now, someone is dead. Here, there are things to be done.

Mrs. Cardone moved to stand beside me and I hugged her, put one hand on her head to guide it to my shoulder. I reached down and put my other hand on Rebecca's hair, stroking it. As Mrs. Cardone sobbed, I looked beyond her to the deep blue lake and the equally azure sky. At the base of their yard, a small dock reached into the water. A red rowboat was tied there and, in the breeze, rocked back and forth, with a faint, repetitive *clink*, on its tether. I wanted to reassure them that the body is only a brief container; that Manny had gone to a better place—and yet, at that precise moment, I couldn't imagine anything more heavenly than what he had just left behind.

Dabbing her eyes, pulling herself together, Mrs. Cardone's resolve seemed composed equally of relief and anger, robbed as she was of the man who had partnered her through more than two-thirds of her life, robbed even of the daily routine that had occupied her for the months of his illness: the bathing, the trips to the hospital, the giving of medications, the nights when he would sleep fitfully, grunting for breath, and she would not sleep at all. Rebecca, dry-eyed, pulled at her grandmother's skirt and demanded a stop to the grieving and help with coloring, a bunch of crayons in her fist—a six-year-old, able to divert all this onto the pages of her coloring book where she could scribble and scratch this mystery away.

Mrs. Cardone straightened. "I'll call my daughter," she

said, then knelt and whispered into Rebecca's ear, scooting her into the kitchen. Next, she directed me. "Call the visiting nurse," she said, "and let her know there's no need for the aide to come tomorrow. I don't want her to make a wasted trip." The death moment, the hard realization, had just passed. We all got busy.

Manny's daughter arrived in the doorway, hesitating, taking in the scene. Mrs. Cardone, the strong one now, held out her arms. "Come to me," she said. "Dad's gone." While they wept anew, I called the visiting nurse, who said, "It's about time. I thought he was going to hang on forever." Then I went into the kitchen to sit with Rebecca.

While Mrs. Cardone and her daughter murmured and talked in the living room, calling friends and neighbors, making the necessary arrangements that keep one from breaking down, from smashing one's fist into the wall, from taking to one's bed, I sat with Rebecca, who said, "*Now* we can color." I colored the birds blue. She colored the flowers and the vines purple and red. She chatted to me about school and about the swimming lesson she took the day before. Death seemed a thing as yet unable to touch her. I wondered if she had a doll somewhere that might later need dressing and feeding, those pretend ministrations and tendings that would prepare her in some way for a day, far in the future, just like today.

I stayed in the kitchen with Rebecca until the funeral home came to collect Manny's body, and his wife and daughter watched as the hearse pulled away. Then

Rebecca and her mother took Mrs. Cardone upstairs to pack a bag—she would stay with them for a while—and I walked out to my car to drive home. Rebecca waved at me from the bedroom window, and I waved back. In a moment she disappeared, but I could hear her as she ran back to her mother and grandmother, laughing, innocent, and alive.

God Bless the Child

~

Cara Muhlhahn, CNM

In every setting where I have seen birth, I have also seen death. No setting can eradicate that possibility entirely—not a hospital, not a birthing center, not home. Anyone who has practiced this career long enough has experienced an infant life extinguish, not because of negligence or malpractice or delivering in the wrong place but because, sadly, babies sometimes die. It's just inevitable.

When I became a certified nurse midwife, I knew intellectually that infant mortality and morbidity would be part of the equation, but I don't think I could have anticipated what it would feel like to look death in the face.

Attesting to the routineness of death, hospital maternity wards have regular morbidity and mortality rounds, meetings to discuss the specifics of cases with bad outcomes. They call it "M and M." But no matter how many times I encounter death, it will never feel routine to me. I will never get used to it. In over 30 years in this field, I still have not been able to accept it as part of reality. It's just so hard to believe that with all of our fetal monitoring devices, sonograms, and excellent prenatal care, we can't prevent infant death. I'm inclined to try to wish it so, but deep down, I know better. Like it or not, life isn't always fair.

Nothing in life really prepares you for the feelings associated with anyone's passing, least of all that of a newborn. I always find myself feeling sad, angry, betrayed, and helpless, whether I am directly involved in a birth gone bad or just on the outside looking in. Like anyone else, I suppose, I struggle to understand all of the factors that led up to death and agonize over whether doing anything differently might have prevented such injustice. But there is no solution and little solace rendered by this seemingly futile exercise.

These days, at every birth, I stand on edge at the moment when the bluish baby comes through the vagina and breathes or doesn't. I never used to feel that way. Until Lilah.

In 12 years and over 500 deliveries in my private practice, I have lost only one baby. It happened in the summer of 2007, and I am still mourning her loss. I may always.

Here's Lilah's story.

LISA WAS MY LAST MOM to deliver before I went on my August vacation. I was headed for Paris for part of the time, Costa Rica for the rest. My son Liam was at camp. I had the luxury of time and the knowledge that there couldn't possibly be a conflict with another delivery, since my other patients had all delivered and I didn't have any more lined up until September. I could spend all the time I needed with Lisa.

She had hired a wonderful, grounded, and experienced doula named Sarah. Sarah had delivered two babies at home, her first in Colorado and the second with me in Brooklyn.

When I went to Lisa's last few prenatal visits, she was completely sick of being pregnant, as most of us are when we go late. It was mid-July, and the heat can be very hard during pregnancy. Legs swell, and sluggishness sets in from carrying around all that extra weight. She was at 41-plus weeks. The baby was moving and a perfect size, presenting head down. But we decided that since she would reach 42 weeks on Monday, instead of going for a routine biophysical then, we would try to get Lilah out before she reached that mark.

We were typically cautious about it. Friday night, I went over and did a non-stress test at home on Lilah, and then we made our plan: I would sweep Lisa's membranes — move my finger around her cervix to separate the amniotic membranes from the lower uterine segment, which stimulates the release of the hormone prostaglandin, which can kick-start labor — and then Lisa would take some castor oil to move things along a little more.

At 7 PM, she took the castor oil. Contractions began

around 10:30 PM I went over early, around 3 AM. I was being very cautious with this baby, mostly because Lisa had been nervous, and her nervousness spoke to me somehow. Her anxiety spread to me.

Which is why I went over to their home way too early—I wanted to calm myself. I listened to the baby when Lisa's contractions were early. They were regular and painful but in the latent phase. By 7 AM, I had listened to the baby for four hours almost continuously, and at that point was feeling ridiculous that we were intervening before the 42-week mark, because everything seemed so great. When labor slowed down a little, I went home to sleep and let Lisa get some shut-eye, too. After a little rest, we would see what her body would do on its own.

Sarah, the doula, went over in the morning and kept Lisa company and in good spirits. They walked around. The contractions were erratic. This didn't worry me. I have had a lot of moms with labors that start and stop over the course of a few days until they finally get going. We call this prodromal labor. If a woman is planning a hospital birth, she is sent home from the hospital to fend for herself when this happens. But not Lisa. She was well attended by her adorable husband, Jordan, her mom, Sarah, and me checking in on her throughout the day, all completely available to her.

I went back to her place around five that evening. We decided to help the baby's head further into the pelvis by wrapping her belly in such a way as to compensate for the baby hanging forward and not really pressing on the cervix. In this way, we might be able to help Lisa to speed things along and get this baby out. Contractions had slowed, so we once more gave her a small amount of castor oil and went for a walk.

By the time we had walked for two hours, Lisa's labor was booming again. We came home, still listening to Lilah's heartbeat. Not a deceleration in sight. And this time, it looked like her labor would keep going. We all took turns supporting Lisa emotionally, with Jordan and Sarah in the lead. I was busy checking Lilah's heartbeat on a regular basis.

Everyone got tired. In home births, we each take a turn helping the mom while others rest. I volunteered to stay with Lisa and support her from about 3 AM until 7 AM. Sarah was lying on a mattress on the floor in the same room I was in. Lisa's mom and hubby were in the other room trying to get some sleep. And valiant Lisa was on her hands and knees during contractions on the bed and lying forward on some pillows or on her side between contractions. Between each bout of contractions, I would place the Doppler on her abdomen and hear the comforting *byk e byk e byk*, 130s and steady. All good.

In the wee hours of the morning, Lisa's water broke with light meconium. Light meconium can mean a lot of things, but in general, to me, it means that I now have to watch the baby more carefully, if that is even possible, and that if I hear decelerations of the heart rate, we should probably consider transferring her to the hospital. We didn't hear any such thing.

When dawn broke, I realized that Lisa had not voided in a while and I could both palpate and observe a full bladder, which is typical if the baby is in an occiput posterior presentation with its head down but facing the mother's stomach. This position is often associated with longer labor, which is what I had been thinking all along. Of course, I have a catheter for that purpose, one that I sterilize for subsequent use. The only problem was that I had sterilized this one really well—so well that it was not patent any longer, meaning it was sealed shut. Nothing could go through it. I tried to cut it down, looking for an open area while still keeping it long enough to function, but no luck.

Lisa had a friend who was going to go to the pharmacy to get another. It was 7-ish, and the pharmacy didn't open until 8 o'clock. I wasn't sure I wanted to wait that long and called my old buddy and colleague Joan. Joan, in her helpful way, asked me if I wanted her to bring one over. I said yes. She did.

Up until then, Lisa's vaginal exams had shown a persistent cervical lip. This is another common finding in an occiput posterior presentation. She had instinctively chosen to be on her hands and knees, a position that would reduce the lip. By the time Joan arrived, with just a touch of pushing, Lisa had rotated the baby into occiput anterior position—with the baby's head facing her back—a more common presentation, often associated with shorter labor. Things began to move forward rather quickly. We emptied Lisa's bladder, and there we were. Joan had brought some fresh energy, Lisa had turned the head into a better position as evidenced by progress of descent, and we were in the pushing stage. We'd turned the corner after a long night of labor.

Lilah came down quickly, as often happens after a stall caused by occiput posterior positioning. Once the baby rotates, things move quickly. I continued monitoring the baby between pushes, which is how I can determine whether the baby is having any difficulty in this stage. It's normal to have some decelerations at this point because of head compression. The bones in the baby's head are being compressed as it passes through the mother's bones on the way out. Deceleration can also occur if there is a cord around the neck. But there were no decelerations. The baby was clearly doing well.

Until we could see three inches of her head gently stretching out the perineum. She then had a deceleration to 60 beats per minute. I didn't like it, and my gut knew that something wasn't right, which was odd, because I have been at deliveries where babies had a lot of those. I had eventually taken one woman to the hospital, where she had hours and hours of those decels, until the doctor finally sectioned her only as a precaution against leaving the baby for hours in a potentially compromising situation. Of course the baby was fine, with a 9-to-10-point score out of a possible 10 on the Apgar scale, which evaluates a baby's heart rate, reflexes, muscle tone, and breathing in the first moments of life. In situations like that, it's hard not to feel as though the mother holds me accountable for an unnecessary Cesarean section.

So here we were on the frontier of triumph, with this one decel. I felt the baby kick. I didn't like it. Lisa felt her kick, too, and said so. I told Lisa we had to get her out *right then*. Lisa pushed like crazy and out she came, still as the night.

I gently told mom and dad not to worry, that a baby who had behaved that well in labor would come around, and I began resuscitating. I had already pulled the oxygen and Ambu bag close within reach before the birth. I was lucky to have Joan nearby, who prepared the Ambu bag and oxygen, while I cleared Lilah's airway. I immediately began resuscitating.

Usually, when I resuscitate babies, they begin to gasp and the heartbeat comes up from less than 60 to over 80 then over 100, and we're out of the woods. Usually breaths alone, either through mouth-to-mouth or from an Ambu bag, result in success. But there was no longer anything usual about this situation.

The resuscitation wasn't working. I gave the Ambu bag to Joan, who kept bagging the baby, while I continued doing chest compressions. The EMS workers who came were unable to help. They tried, but intubation was difficult. All the while, the family was wailing in a way I will never forget. The feeling began—the feeling that I would never be able to forgive myself. Never. It was accompanied by the feeling of *Why me?* Why had everything I had counted on, everything that had worked for the last 20 years, failed? I still don't get it.

I continued bagging and doing CPR in the back of the ambulance all the way to the hospital, but I knew this would end gravely. I mean, how long do babies have before no oxygen to the brain becomes an issue? The official limit used to be considered four to five minutes. Then it was changed to ten minutes. We had passed both of those limits.

Suddenly, all our lives—the parents', the grandparents', the doula's, and mine—were turned upside down. We all started analyzing what we might have missed or could have done differently. We all had to ask ourselves whether this baby would be alive if indeed she had been born in the hospital. And the truth is that we will never know the answer to that question.

EVERYONE GRIEVES UNIQUELY. There is no right way to do it, and we all have a hard time getting through our grief. The level of heartache at the beginning of the grieving process is excruciating, virtually unbearable. It begins to recede only with time. The mental anguish can be overwhelming, too. That part was especially pronounced for me, as the practitioner in this case. I have wracked my brain again and again, trying to ascertain just what went wrong. One aspect of home birth I had never considered before was how hard, emotionally, it is for the midwife when death occurs. There is no team of people with whom to commiserate. The burden of responsibility and understanding falls exclusively on me.

Initially, it was hard not to doubt my judgment about everything. For weeks and months, I revisited every single thought process and action taken over the course of Lisa's labor, and I sometimes do to this day. But, strangely, every time I've questioned myself, people have come out of the woodwork with facts and anecdotes that remind me that I had taken great pains to do everything with proper care.

That very week, a midwife and a physician both told me stories of their losses. The midwife told me about a mom in the hospital who got out of bed briefly to use the bathroom; when she returned to the bed, there was no fetal heart rate on the monitor. One of my backup perinatologists told me about another baby in the hospital who died after being continuously monitored.

Everywhere I turned in despair and self-recrimination, people told me stories that did not support that recrimination. These stories were like a soft wind that spoke gently to me, saying, *You know you did everything to take care of that baby.*

The same thing happened for the parents. Everywhere they went, professionals shared their stories of similar deaths in the hospital. No one exploited the line of thinking that this might not have happened if only the baby had been born in the hospital. And the parents didn't blame me. This sort of grace strikes me as unusual. I am grateful for it.

It was remarkable to me that without knowing anything about what I had been through, people, like angels, appeared to alleviate my sense of blame. I remember one phone call I placed to the state phenylketonuria testing unit. I was telling the woman who answered the phone that their department had attempted to contact Lisa to let her know that one of her baby's PKU results was out of whack and she would need to do a retest. I wanted to investigate whether there was a connection between this wayward lab result and the baby's death.

As I was relating this, the woman said, "Oh I'm so sorry. That must be so hard for you." She was unusually kind, especially considering she didn't know me. I suppose I assumed that because she worked for a state agency overseeing an aspect of birth, she would have felt compelled to pass judgment, particularly since it was a home birth. But no. This woman had had a home birth herself in the 1980s and had nothing but kind words. With a home-birth rate of only about 1 percent, what were the odds that I would be connected with this home-birth–friendly woman on an anonymous phone call to the Department of Newborn Screening?

It felt a lot like someone—God, the forces that be, *someone*—wanted me not to blame myself. These small moments helped me to move gradually toward forgiving myself. They brought me to a new perspective, a bottom-line realization that I can take my responsibility very seriously—and I do—but that doesn't mean that I can always prevent death.

The Changing of
the Seasons

~

Terry Ratner, RN, MFA

THERE ARE TWO main seasons in Phoenix: summer and winter. Our fall and spring are bypassed for long stretches of sameness. Maybe there's a hint of spring in March, when a frail rain falls, casting a silver net over the neighborhood. Then the sky clears and the flowers smell like baby lotion until the aroma is suffocated in blazing heat. These are our seasons.

Nursing also has its own seasons. They follow no direct weather pattern and occur as suddenly as a hurricane or earthquake, without any warning. There are brief periods of calm with little activity, just the daily comings and goings of patients—the ones who recover without much pain, without any scars.

Then the changes occur: Trees with still branches begin their dance; the full moon wears an orange veil as winds throw blankets of dust like confetti up toward the sky. In daylight the air fades to sepia, like an old photograph. That's when code bells chime and intensive care units fill to capacity with dying patients and grieving families. The scent of loss is everywhere, and one can't escape the inevitable season of death.

It begins in the arteries, rushing sounds without words. Some agree, "It's too soon for death." And others welcome the freedom from pain. The season of loss passes by like a series of cold breaths.

THE WAY I PRACTICE nursing might have been different if I hadn't lost my mother in the spring of 1993. The time of year when the nights stay cool and days begin to warm. That's when I began to bond with little old ladies wearing turquoise rings, silver earrings, and glittering beads. I'd hold their hands and laugh with them like old friends. I'd study their faces, searching for a connection: hair the color of freshly fallen snow, skin paper-thin, eyes shining like topaz, and a dimple on the left when they smiled.

My nursing care changed again in the spring of 1999, when my son, Sky, died in a motorcycle accident. All the young patients became a part of me—each one taking up a small space in my heart, trying to fill the emptiness. They brought about poems of music, stanzas without metaphor, making something out of nothing.

It all happened during the season that's sometimes missed. During the season that hides; the one that smells like jasmine and sprouts tulips from the darkness of the earth. A season that cools the evening sky with its sweet resinous wind while orange tree petals drift to the ground like snow. The season filled with colors, of fairy dusters with pink puffs radiating from their centers and clusters of purple wisteria trailing their vines around budding trees. That's the season when my world caved in.

Those deaths affected my career in ways I never understood until now. They left a sickness in my heart that can't be healed with medicine. No chemo, drug, or miraculous homeopathic pill can take it away. No narcotic is strong enough to dull the pain.

My patients are the medicine I need. The elderly ladies with blue hair who want to hold my hand and call me "honey" because no one is with them. The old men with salt and pepper sprinkled on the few hairs they have left telling me a joke because their children are too busy to listen. The young people who are having surgery because they were reckless, the ones I caution and catch myself preaching to—these are the patients that fill my void.

I pre-oped a young man last week. Inside the paisley curtains, he cursed as he shook his head side to side and moaned, sounding more like a pop star singing a song of love and loss than a patient.

"Help me, someone, I can't take this pain any longer," he yelled.

I pulled a chair close to his bed, placed a cool wash-cloth across his forehead, and injected morphine into his vein. I asked him how the accident happened.

"I was riding my dirt bike out in the desert and got carried away performing some fancy stunts. I fractured my left leg."

I looked at the external fixator attached to his leg, the swelling in his ankle and knee, and the metal pins that disappeared in his bone. I watched his temple pulsating and thought about life, about luck, about my son, and wondered why he had to die.

I took his callused hand in mine and listened as he talked about the accident.

"I don't know what happened, the bike just got away from me," he said.

The connection between my patient and Sky went deeper than motorcycles, their bushy eyebrows, big brown eyes, and olive complexion, a build referred to as "buff." I wanted to save this patient from a worse fate. I wanted his parents to be immune to the disease that afflicted me. "You're playing Russian roulette with your life," I told him. I felt his hand squeeze mine. His forehead dripped with tiny beads of perspiration. "My belief is we all die when our time is up. I'm not afraid of death," he said. "We all have to die sometime."

I wanted to put my arms around him and talk about a son who followed that belief. A son who thought he had nine lives and joked about his luck—a son who had two motorcycle accidents before the fatal one. A son who kissed me on the cheek two days before he died for no particular reason. Instead, I told him to be careful. I don't want to burden others with my grief.

Nine years have passed since Sky's death, but the sense of loss lingers, like a potpourri scent that never quite goes away. I want to be reminded of him, of the joys and the heartbreaks. I want to be around others with his interests and language, the gestures that link them as one. And just like a child that grows up and leaves, so do the patients that I connect with. They come and go like the change of seasons — something to count on, like the first rainfall of the year, or the scent of an early bloom leaving us with a bouquet to remember. What remains at the heart of this is its humanity, its search for connections within the seasons of our lives.

Sayonara

~

Lucy May J. Colegado, RN

DEATH WAS CERTAIN, and she implied she was ready.

She signed the DNR form herself, because with stage IV lung cancer, she knew there was no way out. Taking it even further, she requested to be left alone with a nasal cannula, even when her breathing got much worse. She refused the face mask and said that nobody could force her to use it because it was her right to decide what she wanted.

She verbally denied any pain, despite obvious clinical signs that she was in severe or at least moderate pain. She reasoned she didn't want any morphine because it was morphine overdose that had accidentally hastened the death of an aunt and an uncle.

I thought it would be cruel to just watch and not do something. To see a dying patient desperately gasp for air and just stand there was almost unthinkable. I mean, the least I can do is make patients feel comfortable, but if she didn't want to be comfortable and was mentally stable enough to express that desire, what right did I have to impose what I wanted?

I prepared for a long night. I tried to reason and wrestle with my personal demons. I tried to convince myself that death, at this time, must be welcomed.

"Can…you…stay?"

It was 1 AM in the morning and her saturation was on the high 70s. Each breath was a struggle, and her lack of oxygen was beginning to cause panic. I reached for her hand and sat on her bed. Whatever I did to prepare myself for this did not really sink in. I wanted her to stay, and I was scared for her, but I tried to hide it.

"I'm sorry…I'm scared…," I told her.

I told her she didn't have to talk. Not only because talking made her gasp for more air, but also because I realized I was not emotionally ready to wrap up a dead body. Besides, if I were dying and was all alone, I would be extremely scared, too. I didn't even know if any of her loved ones knew that she was dying. All of a sudden, Japan seemed so far away.

I don't know—maybe I was just trying to rationalize my selfish thoughts. Isn't it amazing how selfishness can rear its ugly head even at times of dying?

It was cold, and I was unsettled. She might have been ready, but I wasn't. The irony was chilling.

I sighed when the number started going up. She started to relax and then dozed off. I stayed for a while longer. When I was sure she was asleep, I slowly pulled away my hand, but it woke her up.

"Thank you," she said.

I didn't say a thing, but in my head I thanked her. I wasn't ready, and somehow, for some bizarre reason, she respected that. Or death respected that.

In the morning, I told her I was going and that I had just dropped by to say good-bye. "For the last time," I told myself.

"You'll be back tonight, right?" she asked.

I told her I wouldn't be.

"You're quitting?" she asked.

I told her I would be off for four days and joked that I was not allowed to quit. Then, I was quiet.

She looked away. I assumed she heard clearly, even when the words were left unspoken...

I will not see her when I come back. My good-bye was final.

She reached for my hand, and I reached for hers. I didn't say a thing, but when I gently pressed her hand and she weakly pressed mine back, we both knew we were done with our good-byes.

i marveled.
at the power of touch,
and the power of silence.
i left the room relieved.
the irony was still chilling,
but the certainty of death was almost calming.

Tender Mercy

~

Adrienne Zurub

My FIRST ENCOUNTER with Fallon was on her second trip to our operating room within a 24-hour period. She was intubated and had been unconscious since before her arrival. Her diagnosis during the last week of her pregnancy was idiopathic dilated cardiomyopathy. In simple terms, the stress of extra blood volume to maintain both baby and mother was too much on her heart. Essentially, the shape of her dilated heart contributed to the loss of its functionality, a tragic side effect of the particular drugs Fallon had been treated with before her arrival at Cleveland Clinic. She experienced prolonged episodes of oxygen deprivation to her hands and feet, resulting in her fingers and toes turning black and necrosing.

I heard the entourage coming down the surgical hallway, having just emerged from the close-by elevator. At least ten infusion pumps were stacked in two rows on the steel tree arm, with its metal branches that connected to the bed with the assistance of a hydraulic lift. All the pumps were beeping their calculated pharmacological fluid deliveries. The monitor, not to be outdone, echoed the rhythm of the patient's heart as she traveled down the hallway. The visual details of her heart function demonstrated through frenetic hieroglyphic spikes revealed her diminished cardiac output, the opening and closing of her valves, her heart rate, her pulmonary artery pressure, her body temperature, and the latest cardiac index.

Even the endotracheal tube appeared to pay homage to her; it was delicately poised in her mouth instead of assuming its normal jutting posture. We, the team in OR 50, rolled her gently to the right, inserted the roller device under her, and with a precision move, transferred her and her accoutrements from the intensive care bed to the narrow operating room table.

Once she was on the table, adjustments were made as we acclimated and connected her to monitors, pumps, and the anesthesia machine, and as we recalibrated and titrated fluids, strapped her to the bed, placed electrode dispersive pads, and conducted the rest of the routine operating room procedures. All this was done in preparation for a much deeper sleep under anesthesia so we could proceed with the surgery.

On the long OR table Fallon appeared smaller, more delicate, even though she was weighed down heavily by the tubes, catheters, and numerous intravenous lines hanging like clear spaghetti from the intravenous bags; the intravenous pumps looked like sentries behind her head in the territory of the anesthesia staff.

Someone had forgotten to place the beautiful blue disposable bouffant hat upon her head, so her brilliant brown hair, shiny with youth and perspiration, splashed against the white folded blanket, a makeshift pillow, at the head of the OR table. Naked on the table, she was a vision, and we, her audience, connected with the circumstance of her.

She looked…perfect, except for the chaos that was taking place right beneath her skin. We all took this in before the blue-gray sterile disposable shrouds, the surgical drapes, covered her and then revealed the large gaping hole in her chest.

It seemed so unfair that she was there. It seemed like a big mistake. Even with every pump, IV, and machine foretelling her high acuity and the seriousness of her illness, her gentle age shined so brightly in this OR. I was compelled at that moment to thank the Creator, whoever that might be, for the gifts of my health and the goodness of my family, and to ask him or her to please help me, guide me to give Fallon what she needed from me at that moment. If you closed your eyes for a minute as I did that day in mindful prayer and just listened to the rhythmic sound of her mad heart playing on the monitor, the beeps were comforting in their frustrated attempts to keep going. The human spirit is something else! And in that *brief* gap of prayer for Fallon, my thoughts filled with my mother, who years before succumbed to horrific metastatic breast cancer. And I, the "big time" cardiothoracic surgical nurse on the world-renowned open heart/heart transplant team at Cleveland Clinic, became once again a child.

MY MOTHER DIED AT AGE 52, her new life to start somewhere else, in some other realm. Two days before she died, she called me to drive her to the hospital. I bellyached about it, because I had to go to work. But I took her, and did not realize that *she* knew it was her last ride.

I came to the hospital to visit her the next day and she said, "Is there anything in my urine bag, the Foley bag?" I thought it an odd request, and I said, "No." I am a nurse, but she was my mother! I was a child. So no, I did not notice her kidneys were shutting down. I knew on some level that she was dying, but my mind would not allow for that kind of pain. Not yet.

Mommy looked tired, the way people look when they come home from a hard day at work. She could not eat. She kept throwing up brown liquid bile. I badly wanted her, actually needed her, to eat. I offered her food, demanding that she eat it. My controlled panic was unfolding because somewhere in my being, a child was screaming in fear and panic, knowing what was happening to her.

I seemed to have divided into two or three or four persons trying to deal with the circumstances of her dying. At work I was seeing people die and saving other people, yet I was not able to save her! She was resigned to what was happening to her and at peace with her impending death.

I was so angry at her for leaving me here...alone. But angrier at myself, because with a childish mind, I thought she would last forever. It did not seem possible that she could die and this world would dare continue. I thought that if she died, I would die also.

On her deathbed, she took shallow gulps of air with long intervals between. I am a nurse and yet I do not know what this means, because she is my mother, goddammit!

When my mother died, I crawled into the bed with her and cradled myself into her small, hard space. I touched that space between her top lip and her nose, that grooved ridge of hers with the distinctive tiny holes, so that I would not forget it when I saw her again. Her beautiful hair, that culturally defining mane, jet black with touches of gray, now lay slick on her head, damp with perspiration. She was devoid of smell. Instead, the smells of the stages of death drifted into her room. I whispered in her ear between sobs:

I am like water to you, invisible but needed.
I am like water to you, invisible but needed.
I am like water to you, invisible but needed.

After an uncomfortable time for him, my new husband pulled me away from my mother's rigid body. She died in a corner hospital room on Shaker Boulevard in St. Luke's Hospital. I can still see the window of her room from the street. After her death, I was never to be the same person. Something within me died. I shrunk into myself. I was unable to trust that anyone I loved—my daughter or my new husband—would not be taken away from me. And I loved them more, but showed it to them less.

I was safe hiding within the layers of me. My external mask and the masking ritual of the OR became my shield. Eventually, a trail of Prozac led me out. But I still could not trust this God. No God or Creator that I prayed to could ever deny her life...especially when my mother found her life so late. She was like water to me, invisible but needed. Even in my distance from her, I was close. Always, close.

I was a nurse around all of these world-renowned doctors, surgeons, and healers, yet these professionals could not save my mother. These people, my colleagues, did not ask why my world had ended...they noticed nothing, other than keeping the OR schedule going. The tree leaves still whispered in the earliest part of morning. The morning birds still conversed. And the flesh-plumes of smoke swirled religiously toward the OR lights. The crying, the anger, and the anxiety of my patients were quieted with the push of a syringe delivering liquid satisfaction. At work I religiously worked to save the 70-, 80-, or sometimes 90-year-old patients having their first, second, third, or fourth open heart surgery. Yet my powers were impotent to save my own mother! I felt betrayed. I had betrayed my own mother! I—the one who shone so brightly and the one she allowed to become in life what she could never be—could not save my mother from a painful and frightening death. I grieved.

And then, I grew up.

MY SITUATION WITH FALLON, almost 15 years after the untimely death of my mother, awakened in me first the sadness and then, my overarching need to approach my patient with the greatest dignity and respect. Constantly, my colleagues and I remembered the engulfing sadness that her husband and family were experiencing. Those thoughts and our compassion guided us in our focused efforts to provide Fallon with the very best of our professional skills and talents.

Fallon's appearance was an aberration for us because our patient population tends to be older. Besides, she could have been one of us. She looked so far out of her element. Her body, so graceful on the outside, betrayed the carnage occurring just under her skin, reinforcing the saying that "things are never what they appear to be." Her legs were smooth and on her lower ankle, right above the calcaneus bone, was the most beautifully expressed ivy leaf tattoo, which gracefully circled her small, pale ankle, just above her necrosis and black toes. Ironically, the tattoo was further evidence of her bygone, carefree youth. Her hands, fingers, and nail beds were stark black and stiff from necrosis, yet they were utterly captivating. She had a French manicure with perfectly shaped, white half-moon tips set against her incidental nail beds of black. How striking her hands looked! The contrast of the whiteness of the half-moons of her manicure was articulated beautifully and so serene to behold on her delicate hands.

I held her hand.

In her chart was a neat bunch of spiral notebook papers. On these papers were the written trials and tribulations of Fallon's declining health in this pregnancy. The words were literally drawn in the controlled penmanship of her husband on the wrinkled, worn papers. Her husband vividly detailed Fallon's mysterious and mounting symptoms throughout her pregnancy. He punctuated her progressively failing health with details such as Fallon being unable to simply walk down the stairs. He noted how she complained of being too tired, being in constant pain, and being unable to get up from the sofa in her second trimester. Further, she complained of her hands and feet being cold and numb, her legs were swollen, and she was out of breath…too easily.

There were also the unrequited concerns that they had presented to her obstetrics-gynecology doctor. The documents demonstrated their collective distress and Fallon's growing frustration…with herself *and* her body for not complying with the routine rigors of pregnancy.

This notable scenario crystallizes the urgent need for nurse advocates and a commitment to patient advocacy within all disciplines of nursing. It is difficult to believe that a nurse practitioner, a nurse midwife, or an experienced OB-GYN nurse assessing Fallon across many factors would not have issued a red flag and would have relegated Fallon's concerns and symptoms to routine pregnancy complaints.

I believe that patients in their unconscious state become a conscious entity in surgery, especially during an impending death. I know that they, the patients, are there overseeing the concerted struggle for their life. I imagined Fallon looking at us—at me—doing my best on her behalf. I know she heard the prayers of all of us in the room, both voiced and in silence. With the pronouncement of death, I knew her prayers were answered also.

Within my career as a perioperative nurse, I have witnessed more than the normal instances of postpartum cardiomyopathy threatening or taking the life of the mother, and at times necessitating heart transplantation. Pregnancy, albeit necessary to human reproduction, is undoubtedly a significant stressor on the mother's heart and circulatory system. The heart has to pump increased volumes of blood to the developing fetus as well as sustain the host, the mother. Cases involving some form of maternal-fetal conflict are finally receiving credibility and much-needed research. Cases like Fallon's and those of others provoke (or should provoke) nurses to abandon linear thinking in terms of linkages between pregnancy, heart disease, and idiopathic heart conditions. Fetal imprinting, genomic imprinting, and the evolution of maternal defenses are all areas that are relevant to and impact women's heart health. In this way, we as nurses and advocates are better equipped to inform and educate family, friends, the public...and ourselves.

I WANTED TO HOLD Fallon's blackened hand to my face to awaken in her what was awake in me. Strange. Instead, I held her hand lightly at her right side. How beautiful the French manicure! Some would find it grotesque. But her manicured nails were stunning against the palette of pure black, necrotic nail beds, perfectly shaped white half-moons rounding the tips of her curling, atrophic black fingers. The palm of her hand was still white where the crawling necrosis had yet to work its way up. This was a sight never to be experienced in a lifetime.

We prepared to prep her with surgical soap for the procedure. The removal of the blankets and sheets that covered her in her trip from the intensive care unit revealed the carefree tattoo around her ankle and the initial stages of a blackening of her toes (no manicure). The circular miniature leaf design around her ankle was a residual tell-tale sign of a time when death was not imminent.

I looked into her face and I saw myself and the women I knew. Inwardly (and later alone), I cried for all the women who would not make it even to this point because of some error in diagnosis or an attitude that lessens the severity of a woman's presenting symptoms. I cried because Fallon's diagnosis was a slow, unnerving progression to organ failure and death. And I cried for the women who would die mysteriously and without resolution in the outer reaches of health care.

I do no not have the vocabulary for this
the intersection of two women
in this short sphere of time
giving birth
and dying...
but the beauty in the death of her hands is poignant.
Her French manicured nails
with the semicircle curve at the end of her finger
lay elegantly against the necrotically black nail bed.
Her five fingers deeply blackened.

The weight of Fallon within this OR reminds me of when I observed the *Pietà* at the Vatican in Rome. Mary holding the dead body of Jesus is so beautifully expressed that your body also slumps forward with the imagined weight of it. The heaviness of Fallon both emotionally and physically in that OR was about the same. And the weight and talisman of my experience and the souvenir of her are forever with me.

It Doesn't Have to Hurt

~

Susan Riker Dolan, RN, JD
Audrey Riker Vizzard, RN, EdD

WHEN I FIRST asked my mother, Audrey, to tell me what it was like to be a student nurse over half a century ago, she chose to start by talking about pain. She reminded me that until about the middle of the 20th century, most people died at home. Only gradually did death and dying move to hospitals, where, in a shrunken world composed of an iron bed, a tiny bedside table, and a moveable green privacy curtain, poorly medicated, suffering people waited to die. When she was in nursing school, she said, the medical profession was still emerging from the dark ages of pain control. Morphine was available, but its use was highly restricted. She explains:

As a student nurse in a large city hospital, I took

care of many dying people, most of them in pain. Early in training, students were initiated into a conspiracy of silence: "Never, ever tell a patient he is dying. Never admit that a patient has cancer. Refer all such inquiries to the doctor." However, the physicians, themselves over-worked interns, were no better prepared than the nurses to ease the suffering of dying patients. Nurses knew that to call an exhausted intern snatching a few hours of sleep to come and talk to a patient about death was to risk hearing a roar similar to the response they'd get from poking a sleeping grizzly bear with a sharp stick.

The rationale underlying such secrecy was simple but incredibly flawed: tell patients that they are dying and the shock of the news might kill them! Despite a patient's obvious suffering, we were taught to suspect that the person might be faking it to get more morphine, the only really effective painkiller we had. Therefore, to prevent addiction, regardless of the degree of suffering, most patients were held to the same strict standard: one morphine injection every four hours.

"Breakthrough pain" was a phrase not yet coined to name the pain that surfaces between scheduled doses of pain medications. For those who begged for more frequent relief, we administered a placebo, a shot of sterile saline, while maintaining the fiction that we were injecting morphine. If someone complained too loudly, we might be told to wheel the patient's bed to a room at the end of a long corridor and close the door until it was time for the next morphine shot. Without such a heartless regimen, we were told, patients would surely become addicted. Why addiction was even a concern for a dying person still baffles me.

My mother describes desperate patients who were discovered to have saved and hidden their bedtime sleeping pills for an escape to suicide if the pain became unbearable. When a student discovered a stockpile under a mattress, she was to confiscate the pills and turn them over to the head nurse.

"Looking back, it seems like torture, but no one knew any better," she remembers sadly.

She continues by telling a story about one of her favorite patients:

Because most of our terminally ill patients stayed in the hospital to die, many would lie in residence for months. Students came to know patients well, and we often formed a close emotional tie. My favorite was Carl, a sweet, childless widower. Each morning as I made his bed, he told me stories of his life as a merchant seaman in World War II. On a rust-bucket ship, dodging Nazi submarines, he helped deliver food and munitions to England.

Reading Carl's chart, I learned that although he'd recently survived extensive surgery for colon cancer, no one had told him he had cancer or that the disease had already spread to nearby organs.

Things changed rapidly after his surgery. Each day, Carl became more gaunt as he lost weight and acquired the yellowish skin so typical of such wraiths. Although he suffered constant pain, he rarely complained, and he waited patiently for his shot of morphine. Then one day he asked me to pull the curtain around his bed. "I'm not getting better," he whispered. "Tell me the truth. Do I have cancer?" In those days cancer almost always meant a certain death sentence.

I knew this good man liked me, trusted me, and hoped I might be the one person who would tell him the truth. Nevertheless, as I avoided looking into his sunken eyes, I parroted what I was taught to say: "I don't know. You'll have to talk to your doctor about that." At that moment I believe his long-suffering spirit shattered.

I still recall the shame I felt when I lied to him. But I was a tiny speck in a dust storm of denial. If I broke the rules, I risked getting kicked out of nursing school. Moreover, I was totally clueless as to what I might say to offer him comfort. As a result, he withdrew from me and listlessly turned away when I visited. He died in pain, lonely, hopeless, without human comfort.

Not until the 1960s, when Dame Cicely Saunders smashed the old rules with one sharp bang of her hospice hammer, did things really begin to change. Setting the model for the rest of the world, she founded the modern hospice movement. Her dying patients received Brompton cocktails, concoctions containing liquid morphine, given as often and as generously as needed. Emotional, spiritual, and medical needs were addressed with loving attention.

Despite continuing advances in pain and symptom management, many Americans still die in pain. Patients in hospitals often report moderate to severe pain before dying, while patients receiving hospice care typically report excellent pain and symptom management. Hospice professionals, widely acknowledged as pain management experts, operate with a philosophy that all pain and other uncomfortable symptoms are treatable and everyone is entitled to relief. Nothing is gained by gritting teeth and suffering silently.

Hospice trusts patients as accurate judges of their own discomfort. In assessing its severity, a hospice professional is likely to ask, "On a scale of zero to ten, with ten as the worst pain you've ever had and zero meaning no pain, how do you rate your discomfort?" Then the hospice team works together to address all the patient's needs by gathering detailed information about pain and other symptoms, a history of the disease, current medications, family dynamics, and emotional and spiritual needs.

"What does 'quality of life' mean to you?" a team member may ask before coming up with a treatment plan to meet a patient's needs. One patient or a family member may ask for more medication to ease severe pain while another willingly tolerates more discomfort for the trade-off of being more alert. In extreme cases, a patient or family may request heavy sedation (called palliative or terminal sedation), sometimes to the point of unconsciousness, to escape intractable suffering.

"Tell me the truth," a patient's wife once asked, cornering me, "doesn't hospice really kill people?" Her naked question is not usually expressed so openly, but it lurks in the minds of many. Of course people die while receiving hospice care; however, they die from their disease process, not from hospice care. Hospice care honors a natural dying process while aggressively managing pain and other uncomfortable symptoms.

"Don't use a sledgehammer to kill a flea," advise hospice experts. Wherever possible, hospice starts treatment with small amounts of non-narcotic, over-the-counter drugs, like acetaminophen or ibuprofen. If that works, fine. If not, then they go up the pain relief ladder until they get the desired relief as defined by the patient and caregivers. As a disease progresses, sometimes pain will spike in intensity, necessitating an adjustment in medications.

Not every dying person suffers pain. Not one of my four grandparents died in physical discomfort. Linda was not so fortunate. Early in my career, I visited her home with a hospice nurse to assist with the admission process. Linda's breast cancer had spread to her bones, and she was in severe pain.

Linda's husband, Burt, was a retired physician who had practiced medicine for over 40 years. Now his full-time job was taking care of his wife. Worried and frustrated, Burt told me, "My wife is no wimp. We've managed all right until recently, but now she's crying, complaining of unbearable pain, even as I keep increasing her morphine! She's getting enough to kill a horse but with no relief. What's going on?"

The hospice nurse explained, "Relief from bone pain

requires an over-the-counter nonsteroidal, anti-inflammatory drug like ibuprofen." Given ibuprofen, Linda had significant pain relief within 24 hours. Burt admitted that he had believed the morphine alone would kill any pain. "Pain management was never my specialty," he acknowledged humbly.

Family members often question hospice's use of opioids like morphine. "Won't my loved one become an addict?" they ask. When opioids are used appropriately for pain relief, patients do not become addicts. On the contrary, they gain relief from agonizing distress. Unlike those addicted to drugs, when pain is under control, a hospice patient will seldom request more medication. Nevertheless, tolerance for larger doses of opioids can increase as a disease progresses and pain intensifies. In such cases the hospice team, led by the physician, will adjust doses, switch medications, or try different combinations of potent painkillers until comfort is achieved.

Sometimes a patient who has been on opioids improves enough so that such powerful drugs are no longer needed. Then the team will carefully manage weaning the patient to avoid unpleasant side effects.

My mother told me of an elderly lady who once grabbed her hand and pleaded, "Please, please put a pillow over my head. I want to die!" It's not unusual for someone tortured by unrelieved suffering to beg to die. However, with hospice care, not only can pain be effectively managed, but other uncomfortable symptoms like nausea, vomiting, restlessness, agitation, and difficulty breathing can be brought under control. When such ailments are managed well, the will to live typically returns.

Many people ask about the difference between hospice care and palliative care. Palliative care is intended to ease any type of pain and suffering and is available at any time during a patient's illness. It can be delivered along with life-prolonging and curative treatments. Not all palliative care is hospice care, but all hospice care is palliative, because hospice seeks to bring the terminally ill patient relief from pain and other discomforts. Many hospice programs offer palliative care as a separate service for patients who may need pain and symptom management, although they are not ready for hospice care.

Never Too Late

~

Rachel Shinabarger, RN

I CAN STILL HEAR the sound of her breathing. Gurgling, like the sound of someone drowning.

That's what I recall. Now, I know her lungs were full of fluid. She was drowning and her frail body shook as she struggled to breathe.

As a student nurse on one of my first clinical rotations, all I knew was that this lady sounded horrible, and I was scared. I had already finished giving my first patient his medications and had charted his assessment for the afternoon, and was wondering what to do next. A floor nurse asked me to take in a few get-well cards to the lady I was now sitting next to. This was my second time in that room. The first time, I walked in, shook her gently, and called her name. There was no response, other than the sound of each labored breath. I went immediately in search of her primary nurse to report that something was drastically wrong. I remember the R.N. looking at me as if I were a small child who had asked a very silly question. Well, of course the patient didn't respond: She was comatose; she was a DNR/DNI (do not resuscitate/do not intubate), and her death was imminent. I was not to worry. Just leave her mail by the bed and go help another student. No, we weren't going to suction her; that would just cause more distress. No, there wasn't any family to come in. They were all far away. But they had sent some cards; that was nice. Yes, I should just leave them by the bed and stop worrying. After all, she wasn't responsive anyway. When I asked if I should read her the cards, the nurse just shook her head at me and smiled. Sure, I could read them, but I shouldn't expect her to say thank you.

I walked back into the room and just stood by the woman's bed for a few minutes watching her, her mail still clutched in my fist. I hadn't watched death approach before. Sure, my grandparents had passed away, but I wasn't there to actually see it happen.

This wasn't quiet and peaceful; it certainly was not what I had prepared for. I had imagined myself putting an arm around family as we watched their loved one quietly take her last breath and pass peacefully into another life. This was harsh. There was no one there to grieve her passing; no one to shed tears about a life now finished. No one to whisper in hushed tones about what a marvelous woman she had been, about what a gracious life she had lived and all the people who would miss her. There was no one to tell her she was loved and that it was okay for her to go now. No one except me, and I didn't even know her. I wondered if that would matter. Would she know that I was the only one? Would she hear me if I spoke to her? And did she know she was dying alone? The staff said "no"; she didn't know anything anymore.

Her aloneness washed over me. What if this were my grandma or my mom? I sat on the chair near her bed and opened her cards. I had been taught that hearing was the last sense to go. Would she hear me if I talked? They were get-well cards from family and friends, just a few. I read them aloud to her and then sat silently. What else was I supposed to do? I looked around, feeling rather foolish, but then I started to talk. I told her that her family missed her and that I was a student nurse and didn't have a clue what I was doing. I told her about how scared I was and how afraid of failing. Did she hear me?

Then I told her about the beautiful fall day just outside her window. How blue the sky was. How the trees were all scarlet and gold with leaves just starting to drift on the breeze. I told her about the huge white powder-puff clouds in the sky and how I always wanted to jump from cloud to cloud when I was a child, just like in the stories of Raggedy Ann. I whispered her name and squeezed her hand. I told her it would be okay. She didn't need to be scared now. I would come back tomorrow and sit again. And then I felt the slightest pressure on my hand. This woman who I was told could not respond squeezed my hand, ever so slightly, but the response was so very real.

Startled, I looked up at her face. Her eyes remained closed and her lungs still rattled as she struggled for every breath, but there were tears rolling down her face. I simply sat with her then.

Eventually, my instructor came in then and told me it was time to go. There was other work to be done. I went back the next day to see the woman as I had promised, but the room was empty. She had died during the night. I walked back to my car, thinking how fragile life is, and then my tears came: tears for someone's mother and wife, grandmother and friend, dying alone. And tears that maybe, just maybe, I had touched her in those final moments, and she knew that someone was with her, that she was not alone.

I realize that some might say the hand squeeze was reflex movement, or that I had imagined it. Perhaps that's so. But the tears were real, and I believe that for just a few minutes, she was given a gift: a moment of clarity in which she heard me call her name and knew that I cared. I've been a nurse for 15 years now, and the dying process is still difficult for me to watch, though I no longer find it so scary. But I have never forgotten that woman and what I learned from her. It is never too late to make a difference in someone's life. Even in our final moments, comfort and care can be given and received.

A Nurse's Recovery
from Grief

~

Keith Carlson, RN

As a nurse, illness and death naturally run like a subterranean current through my professional life. Patients struggling with AIDS, cancer, and chronic illness have entered and exited my life for more than a decade, leaving indelible marks. The nurse–patient relationship frequently elicits emotional intimacy when the chemistry is right, and the bonds that I've shared with some patients and families have often been moving and personally transformational. Being present for an individual's dying process is an intimate privilege — and one that I do not take for granted. Death is a natural part of life's trajectory through which we all inevitably must pass, and nursing has afforded me authentic glimpses into the raw emotion that death can elicit.

In my professional life, I have comforted the sick, the dying, and the grieving. The strong emotions experienced in my role as a nurse have occasionally brought me great sorrow, and I have grieved the loss of many beloved patients. My professional experience certainly has assisted me in being present for friends and loved ones in their moments of illness, loss, and grief. In my personal life, multiple losses and my own grieving process are quite distinct from—yet informed by—my work as a nurse.

Between 2001 and 2008, I lost four beloved beings in my circle of intimate family. Over the course of less than seven years, these four significant and singular individuals left this earthly existence, and my grieving process in the wake of those multiple losses is at times as fresh as it has ever been. I continually navigate these waters of grief, and although there are many helpful navigational tools within easy reach, the journey is one that ultimately we all must take alone. It is a journey born of loss, and the learning therein is indeed grist for the mill as we all experience the lives, loves, and losses that life brings our way.

In 2001, not long after the events of September 11th, a dear family friend entered a New England church on a sunny winter morning in search of political asylum. Verbalizing fears of government surveillance of his political activism, he described being questioned and followed by federal agents the prior evening. After an exhausting and sleepless night, he entered the church, threatening suicide with a knife if his request for protection was not heeded. Tragically, misinformed and hypervigilant policemen rushed the church and startled my friend, riddling his body with seven bullets within a minute of their entry, despite the fact that he had made no threatening movements toward anyone but himself. He died an agonizing death, and we were left with the cruelty of a sudden and unexpected loss brought about by unnecessary violence. His loss reverberates through my immediate family to this day, and my wife, my son, and I still reel from the reality of his absence. He was our family confidante and playful friend, an anchor for us all. He had a special and distinct friendship with each of us, and we each felt his loss keenly, and do so to this day. Grief and post-traumatic stress visited us on that day in December 2001, and its pall is yet to fully disperse.

Some three months later, I lost yet another close friend. My great-aunt—a well-known painter—died at the age of 115 following several years of mental and physical decline. At her advanced age, death was not unexpected, yet she had been lucid and active until the age of 112, publishing books, selling paintings, and regaling us with stories of her life that touched three historically significant centuries. Her death marked the end of an era for me. It was the loss of a great friend, a mentor, a teacher, and a beloved family member whose driven life of purpose and determination served as a beacon to us all.

Several years passed before another major loss hit me like an engulfing wave. Sparkey was a dog like no other. His companionship and boundless loyalty were like balms to my soul, and as he aged and grew ill, his impending loss began to overtake our family. Being a nurse, I assumed the responsibility for administering daily IV fluids to stave off the ravages of renal failure. When he became skeletal and weak, with eyes pleading for an end to his suffering, we chose to have Sparkey leave his old body as he lay on one of his favorite beds on our screened-in porch, his beloved perch for watching the world that he loved go by. A vet administered the medications to gently ease him from his body as my wife, my son, and I sat by his side. As he began to slip into unconsciousness, he gently licked each of us on the face, a sweet final act of gratitude that was followed by a single tear falling from his right eye before both of his eyes closed forever. After spending some time with his poor wracked body, we buried him in our yard in one of his favorite spots. A dogwood bush and three rhododendrons now grow abundantly there, and perennial flowers planted by our son in Sparkey's memory poke their hopeful heads toward the sun each spring as tangible reminders of the vibrant and miraculous cycles of death and rebirth.

Last but not least, my 80-year-old stepfather—diagnosed with pancreatic cancer six months before Sparkey's death—steadily declined as 2006 ended and 2007 began. Several hundred miles away yet held close in my grieving heart, he and my mother became a major life focus for myself and my two siblings and our spouses, and we all devoted great stores of energy to their care and support. We leaned in even more closely as treatments failed and death neared, my wife and I eventually taking leaves of absence from work to be at his side. As anticipatory grief gripped our family, I assumed a central role in orchestrating his palliative care. Exactly one year and a day following Sparkey's death, my stepfather took his last breath as we bade him farewell, my mother blessing him with her love and promises to continue on in his absence. It was the fourth loss of this decade for me, and it was a blow that brought me to my knees, both spiritually and emotionally.

Grief can settle in many places in the body and mind. It can insinuate itself at work, at home, and at any intersection of an individual's emotional life and the outside world. Grieving is an elongated process that can take one by surprise, rising again and again to the surface at the most unlikely of times, often just as one feels that some progress has been made. There are physical, emotional, psychological, and spiritual manifestations of grief and mourning, and it is this all-pervasive aspect that makes it so keenly universal. In my own personal universe, chronic pain, new health problems, burnout, and "compassion fatigue" at work all rose to the surface. I was forced to examine my life quite closely, take steps toward change, and implement strategies to decrease stress and simplify my life. It was an all-out effort to survive and to remain plausibly functional in both my personal life and my demanding professional capacities.

The keen sense of loss that became part and parcel of my internal process rendered me more sensitive to others' losses in the long term, and that has indeed served me well in my professional life. Still, the stress and illness brought about by my grieving and mourning eventually wore away at my ability to be fully present for others as a nurse, and that was a clear indication of the need to focus in closely on my own emotional health.

Although I acknowledge Elizabeth Kübler-Ross's crucial identification of the stages of grieving, I have come to see grief as a vast continuum along which the individual travels from moment to moment. Throughout my grieving process, I have yet to identify a single static "stage" that I have traversed. Rather, my grief is more like an ocean in which I swim, and the amount of support and buoyancy that I require at any given moment varies quite wildly. Indeed, there are times when the grief seems to have dissipated entirely, and thoughts of my departed loved ones pass over my mental screen with nary a ripple of pain. At other times, the pain of loss can come to the forefront without warning, stopping me in my tracks and pinning my shoulders to the mat as I strive to navigate what had just moments before seemed like an ordinary day. Grieving is a constant mystery that is filled with surprises, and one must simply prepare for such surprises as best as one can given the available tools of survival at hand.

There are many tools that I have found helpful, and one of the most profound tools in my grieving toolbox is writing. Through the written word, in both public and private formats, the processing of my emotional life has been incredibly therapeutic. Telling my story, honoring my departed loved ones, sharing the details of my emotional life, and using words to impart my experience provides a therapeutic outlet that not only meets my needs, but also shares it with others as they experience their own lives and losses. Words can be healing, as much for the writer as for the reader.

Psychotherapy is another tool that has helped to move my grieving process along. The therapist is an objective witness to my pain who can also offer me survival strategies and has been a gift that I have freely given myself for several years. This sacred and trusting relationship buoys me in times of distress and affords me time strictly devoted to my own self-care and healing. Rather than a sign of weakness and poor coping, I see allowing myself such a level of self-nurturance as a sign of personal strength, of recognizing and honoring my own deep need for unconditional acceptance and support.

There is nothing like movement and exercise to assuage mental suffering. Despite chronic pain that at times hinders my ability to exercise as much as I would like, the active use of my body offers an escape wherein my mind can let go and I can simply be in the moment. As I swim, walk, stretch, or practice yoga or Qigong, my mind can sink down into my body and I enter the present moment in a new way, refreshed and temporarily relieved from the "busy-ness" of the mind. Science has shown us that exercise causes the release of endorphins and other antistress hormones. There have been moments while swimming that I have entered a world in which neither pain nor stress exists, and those moments are truly gold for the mind beset by grief, loss, and the deleterious effects of stress.

The mind is where thoughts and stress originate, and it is also here where we can learn skills to short-circuit the negative patterns that bring us distress. The practice of mindfulness and meditation are the newest tools that I have introduced to my regimen of recovery. Using mindfulness, conscious breathing, and guided meditation, I am working to more actively focus my mind in the present moment, developing a way to "witness" my suffering without necessarily "being" my suffering. Teachers such as Pema Chodron, Jon Kabat-Zinn, H.H. The Dalai Lama, and Thich Nhat Hahn offer practices that allow one to sink into the breath and witness one's thoughts and feelings without attachment.

Meditation and mindfulness are not necessarily about stopping the thinking process. They simply present strategies that allow a process of stepping back from one's thoughts, witnessing them like clouds passing across the sky. The thoughts are there, but a choice can sometimes be made to allow them to simply move across the mental screen. My own ability to put these principles into practice is still a work in process, although I am currently making positive inroads that I believe are taking me in the healthiest possible direction — toward emotional wholeness and self-acceptance. At times, mindfulness simply means that I acknowledge and gracefully accept that I feel bad in the moment, that grief has overtaken me, and that my feelings of loss are overpowering. Frequently, mindfulness is simply being mindful of the presence of pain.

Tools or no tools, my grieving process is just that—a process. As a process, it is elongated, tangential, and circuitous, and it is riddled with potholes and bumps that can challenge me along my path of personal recovery. Friends, family, gifted professionals, and colleagues assist me in my attempts to continue to care for myself in ways that honor my grief and trust my inner sense of right action. There are moments of great self-doubt, but there are also moments of feeling that grief is not forever, and even in the setting of my dear friend's murder by overzealous police officers, there is indeed room for forgiveness and closure, even if my emotional train has yet to arrive at that particular station.

Loss is unavoidable in this life, and since time began, human beings have navigated these troubling waters. While I hope not to sustain further major losses anytime soon, life is anything but certain, and I hold fast to the awareness that those closest to me will someday depart this life—either slowly or precipitously—and that there will never be a "good" time for such an experience. Nonetheless, at this point in my own journey I can see that I have evolved with each loss, and the Herculean work of grieving has caused me to grow and stretch in ways previously unforeseen.

My work as a nurse frequently brings me into contact with those facing or recovering from major loss, be it the loss of life, of a loved one, of wellness, or of independence. My own losses and experiences of grief inform my ability to be present for those I encounter under such circumstances, and I bring to bear my own personal treasury of learning from navigating these turbulent but inevitable waters. The faces of my own departed loved ones frequently come to mind, and as I recall the gifts that they gave me—both in life and in death—I give thanks for the opportunity to have known and loved them, despite the pain of letting go again and again, and I can truly say that it is indeed "better to have loved and lost than never to have loved at all."

She Inspired Me

~

Irma Velasquez-Kressner, RNC

SHE IS NO longer with us; she is in heaven sharing her kindness with many other angels. I met "Bette" when I was her nurse at a telemetry unit. Her face and smile constantly conveyed kindness and love. Bette was not only a beautiful human being, a devoted wife, mother, and grandmother; she also was a eucharistic minister at a Roman Catholic Church.

I worked 12-hour shifts and I rarely did three days in a row, but this time I had the privilege of taking care of Bette for three consecutive days. She was appreciative of any little thing I did for her and was delicate and polite whenever she had a request.

Bette was a 68-year-old lady who had suffered rheumatic fever as a child. It compromised her heart valves, and she consequently developed congestive heart failure.

Being at the end-stage of her condition, she was on a continuous dobutamine drip, a positive inotropic agent used for the treatment of CHF. She had great support from her husband, who was taking care of her IV port, changing her dressings, and replacing the medication bag when it was empty.

Bette had asked her cardiologist about her prognosis when she started on the medication. As she explained to me, the physicians told her that in most cases medications extend the patient's life for about three to six months. When I first met Bette she had been on the drip for over six months. "She is an angel on earth" is what I figured soon after.

At the end of my shift and on the third day, I said good-bye to Bette, and she handed me an envelope with a note that read:

Irma,

My family and I truly appreciate your friendly manner and expertise. I definitely lucked out being in your care these 3 days. You're a part of a great team. The PCU team and I Thank God I'll be going home because of all the efforts extended to me.

Please take care of yourself because we need your kind of health care and you have to have the strength and health to go at the constant rate you work.

My mom was a smart woman. She always

said, "Good things come in small packages." She was right!!!

God Bless you,
Bette

This note deeply touched my heart. I did not know at this point that this beautiful and gratifying experience was just starting and that it was going to become the most memorable of my career.

A couple of weeks later, Bette was readmitted to our unit. She told me that she was planning a party to celebrate her life, and wanted to know if I would be able to attend. She was grateful to have outlived the statistics of patients who were on a dobutamine drip for more than six months. Bette invited a couple of nurses from my unit, her cardiologist, her medical doctor, and many friends and family members. Her invitation said:

The year 2003 is rapidly coming to an end and I have many to thank and praise for supporting me through the many medical challenges and technologies I have faced these past couple of years. The Almighty God, my loving family, great doctors, caring nurses, wonderful friends and sincere Ministers of Eucharist. All blended to extend my life this year.

And so it's payback time—and maybe more months, more years, more miracles will come my way.

In the meantime and while preparing for her party, Bette was admitted into my unit more and more often. If I was not her nurse, she asked for me and requested that I come to her room to say hello. She always appeared so happy to see me, showing an instant, beautiful smile full of kindness. Yet I was saddened each time I heard that she was back to my unit, because I knew that her condition had deteriorated.

Bette's orthopnea did not allow her to sleep flat, so her neck was often sore from sitting up. In an effort to relieve the tension in her neck, I rolled a couple of towels and secured them with surgical tape. She loved my "invention," and it became her favorite "security blanket." Each time she was admitted, she would request that I make it for her, and she would comment to her family how much she loved "the neck roll that Irma made for me."

One morning I had an amazing and privileged experience that I will always treasure. When I heard that Bette had just been admitted to our floor, I came to say hello. She was sitting on a reclinable chair, talking on the phone. I stood outside, waiting for her to become available. She turned her head, gave me her beautiful smile, and shouted on the phone, "My angel is here. I have to go!" She immediately hung up the phone and greeted me.

A real angel was calling me her angel. What a privilege! What a reward!

Bette never protested about her medical condition or misfortune. She always had a positive attitude and never took anything for granted. She was compliant and accepted her situation, and was making the best of it. Every day was a blessing for her because she knew she had been given the gift of living longer than medically expected.

Soon after this, as she was being admitted to the hospital so frequently and returning home with minimal improvement, Bette told me, "I don't want to do this to my family anymore. I will just stay home and I am trying to make arrangements for a visiting nurse and home hospice."

Bette had always asked me to call her to say hello when I had a chance. I had refrained from doing this, because I knew that it was unethical while she was my patient in the hospital. Now that she was no longer going to be admitted, I started calling her at home.

She was always so happy when I called her, and occasionally she called me. One winter morning, I called Bette. While we were talking, she said to her husband as he walked into her room, "Oh, my God, the sun just came out! It was so dark and cloudy, and Irma called and the sun came out; did you see this? She busts me up with energy and lights up the room!" This was another beautiful and rewarding moment, receiving a compliment from my dear patient, that I will never forget.

Bette's party was postponed by a severe storm the day of the event, and she had to reschedule it for two months later. She wrote a letter apologizing to everyone for the delay. By the time the party took place, she had been on a dobutamine drip for 13 months. It was a great pleasure to be part of her party. She was wheeled to the room looking debilitated but with a large and angelical smile. She was full of love, pride, and tenderness. The room was filled with people who loved and admired her deeply.

Among many speakers, there was a couple who sang and played the violin as they dedicated a song to Bette: *"You raise up so I can stand on mountains/You raise up to walk on stormy seas/I am strong when I am on your shoulders/You raise me up to more than I can be."* While listening to the song, I looked at Bette, who looked humble and proud at the same time. I realized how fortunate I was to have come across such a beautiful human being.

I was not surprised to see how many people loved and admired her. I remember how many times her compliments and appreciation had "raised me up so that I could stand on mountains" and be the best I could as a nurse. I realized the great effect she had made on me as a nurse and as a person. As the song says, "she raised me up to more than I could be." I had never heard this song before and to this day, I have tears in my eyes each time I hear it. I later purchased the CD, and I play it when I have a difficult day at work or when the challenges of my profession become overwhelming. Bette's song always raises me up.

Two other nurses attended the party, and together we got her several items that we thought would make her life more comfortable at home, including a real neck roll, special pillows, and bed raisers. Bette called me at work the next time I was in and thanked me for the gifts. Once again she was "raising me up" with her compliments. Soon after, I received this thank-you card in the mail:

Irma, Irma, Irma!!

You are incredible! Not just as a nurse, not just as a friend, and not just as a person. You put me to shame. You are the most giving person I know. Your energies touch so many lives and feelings. I am truly overwhelmed! I knew you were SPECIAL the first day I met you. You were sent by God to me when I needed care and encouragement the most. Your vibrant energy, humor and laughter lift up my spirits. I am so comfortable in your care...I love your accented voice and sweet words you use to address all of us "Darling." That's what you are, a darling, darling lady. Your daughter is a very lucky lady—Elliott too.

You are a treasure and thank God for you especially at this time of my life!

Love you, Bette

It had been more than a month since Bette had decided to remain at home and about a week since the party celebrating her life. She called me at the hospital to ask if I could make her the "neck roll," saying her husband would pick it up. Though we had given her a real one at the party, she wanted the one I made.

I visited Bette at her home once after this, and I also called her every so often. She continued to deteriorate, and I noticed the weakness in her voice on the phone. She started planning her funeral, including the songs to be played at the service. One day when I called, her husband told me that she was very weak and too tired to talk but that she sent me her regards. I became concerned and asked him to call me if she felt like talking or if I could be of any help. Two days later at work, I saw Bette's medical doctor standing at the nurse's station. "Our Bette is not doing so well," I said to the physician, who sadly replied, "She passed away yesterday."

I felt a terrible sadness and emptiness in my heart; I had to go to another room to cry and to compose myself. The angel who thought I was her angel passed away on Easter Sunday, surrounded by her children and grandchildren. She had become a miracle who outlived the statistics. She survived for 14 months with a cardiac drip that has allowed other patients to live only an extra three to six months.

I attended her wake that night after work. She looked beautiful, kind, and peaceful—just as she always had. I have kept in touch with her husband, and my husband and I have invited him to our house for the holidays.

Bette will always be my inspiration to continue to do what I love: taking care of patients while giving the best I can. Being a nurse is a privilege that overshadows our challenges, frustrations, and adversities. Being a nurse and having experiences like the one I had with Bette helps me to disregard the frequent misconceptions of the public and the media about what we nurses really do.

Lessons from Our Patients

~

Karen Kupsco, RN, CHPN

As a child, I was always fascinated by the field of nursing. I would devour books with registered nurses as the main characters, but I never felt that I could make their world my reality. Sadly, it was something quite simple that made me feel that way: an aversion to needles.

When I graduated high school and chose to pursue a degree in Special Education, I felt as if I were settling for a career that didn't speak to my soul. However, when I pictured what I thought nursing school would entail (practicing starting IVs on and giving injections to fellow students, and having the same performed on me), I vowed to complete my studies and become a teacher.

In my thirties, having left college to marry, I began to contemplate what my future would hold. My children were of school age and reasonably self-sufficient, and I longed to return to a formal learning environment. My grandmother, at age 92, was experiencing a recurrence of breast cancer, having undergone a radical mastectomy and enjoyed five symptom-free years. Sitting at her bedside, I was present for a visit from her hospice nurse. My grandmother was visibly weaker, and asked the nurse bluntly, "When will I die?" I expected platitudes and reassurances, the comment that she would be fine. Instead, the nurse replied, "You're not ready to die yet, but I'll be here with you. I'll tell you when it's getting closer so that you can prepare."

At that moment, the seed of love for nursing, which had lain dormant for so long, took hold. I vowed to do whatever it would take to enter the field of nursing, to be rewarded with the privilege of interacting with patients the way my grandmother's nurse did: with compassion, kindness, and honesty.

I was pleasantly surprised to learn that nursing school did not, after all, involve experimentation with needles. We practiced on manufactured, pliable, and cooperative body parts, honing our skills until we were ready to use them on human beings. My years in nursing school passed quickly, and despite there being few hospital nursing positions open to new graduates, I was fortunate to be hired as a night-shift RN on the Oncology floor at Alexian Brothers Medical Center in Park Ridge, Illinois.

The night is the scariest time for the sickest patients, and I felt ineffective because I did not have the time between administering medications and completing paperwork to sit at their bedside and comfort the frightened and dying. I was disheartened as I observed patient after patient being subjected to chemotherapy when it was obvious that the opportunity for aggressive treatment had passed. I grieved for their inability to find the strength to say "enough is enough" to their families and resented physicians who did not present that choice. I felt strongly that in many cases, these patients could enjoy a more comfortable, peaceful time as death neared, one spent with loved ones at home actively preparing for their journeys from their earthly lives. I longed to be the kind of nurse that cared for my grandmother: a hospice nurse.

Once hired as a hospice nurse case manager, I began my training and became increasingly comfortable in my new field. Although overwhelmed at first, I quickly became acclimated to the new pace and focus of hospice nursing. One of my first patients, Anthony, had been a pediatric dentist, one of the pioneers in his field. He loved his work passionately and lived to practice, working long after his diagnosis of colon cancer until excruciating pain and weakness forced his retirement. I was privileged to build a relationship with him, and ensured that he remained comfortable as his condition declined.

I vividly remember a Friday afternoon visit, during which his son was at the bedside. As Anthony's level of consciousness and functionality had deteriorated so rapidly that week, I was shocked to find him sitting up in bed when I arrived, pen and paper in hand, instructing his son about funeral planning (including choosing each song that would be played and supplying CDs) and various financial and practical issues. I was amazed to see him so alert, speaking in such a strong voice. My acute-care nurse's heart didn't see what my newly minted hospice heart would soon know.

I attended a gathering for my interdisciplinary team that Friday evening. While speaking about our patients, I happened to share Anthony's name with our team chaplain, Gina. I was amazed to learn that he had been her dentist as a child. Now, in her thirties, Gina still remembered his kindness and the way he had made a little girl feel so comfortable, cared for, and relieved of fear. I smiled, anticipating sharing that story with Anthony, knowing how much it would mean to him to know that he was remembered so fondly after so many years.

Although tempted to pick up the phone and call him immediately, I waited, thinking I had plenty of time to do so because Anthony had appeared so much stronger earlier that day. As I was leaving the party, I picked up my cell phone to call Dr. M, eagerly anticipating sharing Gina's comments. His wife answered, breathless, asking, "Are you coming?" Anthony had just taken his last breath.

As I completed his post-mortem care, I grieved having lost the opportunity to let my patient know, at the end of his life, how much his kindness, compassion, and skill had meant to a little girl, now grown up. As I looked into his peaceful face, I learned my first hospice lesson: Never postpone or overlook an opportunity to share positive thoughts. I vowed from that moment to always be attentive to the lessons that my patients would teach me and to always trust my heart and my instincts.

Mel's Story

~

Pato Cog, RN

I PRACTICE THE ART of nursing by ministering to those who are facing terminal illness. I am not a person who has been trained as a registered nurse and who now works in hospice; rather, I am a hospice nurse. What might once have been a job, a career path, or even an interesting diversion is now woven into the fabric of my being: It is my purpose. I have come to know this because of the people I have encountered as my patients and their families.

In the book *Bridges Not Walls*, a text on interpersonal communications, editor John Stewart cites two basic assumptions: 1) "the quality of each person's life is directly linked to the quality of communication he or she experiences," and 2) "there is a basic movement in the human world, and it is toward relation not toward division."

These two ideas can be demonstrated within the interactions of all my patients/families and me. It was, however, one of these particular patient/family encounters that provided for me the epitome of Stewart's two assumptions and changed hospice from ever being merely my work.

My primary professional role at that time was to be the first person at the home scene from the patient-care team. I would perform the initial assessment. This usually consisted of collecting a brief overview of the patient's history, completing a physical exam of the patient, addressing any immediate clinical issues, and identifying any psychosocial needs that might present themselves. I usually spent a significant amount of time with the family, allowing them the opportunity to "tell their story," which generally seemed to be therapeutic. I also would reiterate information regarding the hospice services available to them. I acknowledged that they might be feeling overwhelmed by this information, and that any concerns, questions, and requests for clarification were welcome as any time, 24 hours a day. This often helped to create a trust relationship with our organization, for which I felt a great responsibility and that I strongly valued. In retrospect, I think I had rather unconsciously thought at that time that I was there to give support, caring, and comfort to those in need, and had paid little attention to what I might be receiving from these interactions.

Mel was a 72-year-old man diagnosed with prostate cancer that had metastasized to his lungs and bones. He had responded well to chemotherapy and radiation treatments until the previous week, when he required hospitalization for sudden development of pain after the conclusion of a chemotherapy cycle. His history also included previous myocardial infarctions. During this recent hospitalization, it was determined that his weakened heart could not tolerate further chemotherapy treatment, so hospice was offered to shift the focus from curative to intensive palliative care.

His wife, Donna, was noticeably younger than he, closer to my own age. We met and talked in the kitchen downstairs, while Mel was sleeping upstairs. Donna was an attractive, well-educated, caring woman who was very aware of the gravity of her husband's condition. Perhaps because of the closeness in age, I could easily identify with her and our conversation became more casual. At my invitation, she told me how they had met: She had been recently separated at the time, a single mother with three young boys to raise, and her role brought her to senior citizen groups, presenting informational seminars. Mel apparently had attended one of Donna's presentations reluctantly, at the persistent urging of his sister, but found himself paying attention with a very different interest. He approached Donna afterward, and with courteous restraint, politely expressed his personal interest. Donna laughed at the recollection, remembering her surprise and confusion. As they talked together, Donna realized how truly kind and sincere this man was, and so explained that she was currently going through a divorce and couldn't really think about dating at the time. He asked when she *could* think about it, and randomly she said "in six months." Donna said that exactly six months later, Mel called her and again asked for a date. She said that then she agreed and they began to see each other.

She reflected that as their relationship was developing and Mel proposed marriage, she would lovingly, yet with some real fear, tease him about his age and past heart attacks, saying, "Oh, sure, we'll get married and then you'll have a heart attack and leave me!" She said Mel would respond good-naturedly to this and assure her that he would give her at least 20 years, after which she'd probably be glad to be rid of him. She disclosed this last ruefully; they had been married just three years when Mel became terminally ill with cancer.

We went upstairs to their bedroom where Donna introduced me to Mel, who was now awake, and I performed the requisite physical examination. Mel was alert and oriented, though bed-bound by his extreme weakness and fatigue. I was struck most by the interpersonal communication between Mel and Donna. They looked and spoke to each other in a way that expressed their obvious mutual love in a subtle yet powerful manner. I felt energized to be in the same room, their love was so palpable. The betweenness so often mentioned in *Bridges Not Walls* was in observable action for me that day. During my learning of this phenomenon of betweenness, I would return in thought to that afternoon with Mel and Donna, noting it as my frame of reference for this concept of what occurs between people outside words as they communicate.

It was five or six weeks later when I was called to see Mel again. I don't usually have the chance to return to visit a patient. My role was to conduct the initial assessment visit, which sets the stage for my peers—the patient-care team—to follow. This first visit is generally my only contact. Apparently Mel's regular nurse had been unavailable to see him, so I was being asked to do a check-in visit. I remember it as a beautiful Friday, late afternoon. I had completed my work for the day (a rare occurrence) and was looking forward to getting off an hour early. Because of this, I was none too happy to receive a last-minute assignment, especially one outside my accustomed duties. Further, I didn't realize immediately that it was Mel that I was asked to see. I was given his last name in this extra assignment, and because it had been several weeks since I had done his original assessment, with my having seen many patients since, I didn't even remember if I had ever met this person. Once I did register where I was going, my attitude shifted. I looked forward to seeing Mel and Donna again, yet I had no idea of the gift that I was about to receive.

Upon my arrival, Donna greeted me warmly and ushered me to the living room, where we sat facing each other on the couch. I recall her exact words: "I have to tell you what's been going on for the past two weeks before you go up and see Mel." She proceeded to report what could be interpreted as a bizarre story, yet her voice was calm and even peaceful. I listened.

Donna said that Mel had really declined since my

first visit and his pain had escalated significantly, requiring frequent titrations of morphine. Setting the scene, she then said that a few weeks earlier, in the middle of the night, she heard Mel's voice. His hospital bed was in the same room as their bed so Donna would be near if Mel called out at night. At first she thought it was Mel beginning to hallucinate from the pain medication. "But then I listened," she said, and it sounded like a completely lucid conversation. She called to Mel, asking if he needed something. He answered kindly and calmly, "I can't talk to you now, I'm busy. I'll talk with you in the morning." Donna was flabbergasted and confused by this response and felt helpless. In the morning when she asked Mel about the episode, he commented with clarity and alertness, saying, "Surely you must know that I'm living in two worlds now. Those people you heard me speaking with last night are helping me make my transition."

These words of Mel's sent a chill through me. This was a belief system that was developing in my own mind, but I couldn't exactly verbalize its rationale with satisfaction. Now, here, Donna was telling me that Mel experienced evidence to support such concepts. Renowned philosopher Martin Buber observed that "the human person needs confirmation… It is from one to another that the heavenly bread of self-being is passed."

Donna went on with her fantastic story by saying that in the days to follow, the most amazing events continued to unfold. Mel had become so weak that he could no longer even turn in bed without help. Further, he had not been eating at all. One day Donna came into their bedroom to reposition her debilitated husband. She found him sitting up independently in bed, gesturing as if he were eating and drinking. Donna was astonished at this sight, asking Mel what was going on. He replied, "Oh, we're having a party," and named foods and beverages with relish that had been favorites of his in the past and were present at this party. Donna was ready to assign this to hallucination, yet she said that in the following days, Mel would speak clearly and coherently to her of what he could see and experience during the visits with "these people."

He told Donna that sometimes it was as if he could see the future, with her and the boys remaining behind after he had left his body completely, and that all would be well for them in his absence. He tried to reassure and comfort her as he explained the visions he had of his future, of how beautiful it was going to be. He would tell her that there were really no words to describe such scenes, that she would just need to believe him, as he believed his visitors.

Then Donna spoke of her youngest son's incredible response to these unprecedented happenings. Apparently, nine-year-old Douglas asked his mother tentatively if Mel was really talking to dead people. Donna believed in the need to be honest, even in the presence of these unconventional behaviors, so she told her son that yes, that's what seemed to going on. He responded with relief and asked sincerely, "Well, then is it all right if I ask him to say 'hello' to Grandma?"

Donna was thunderstruck with his reaction. She took this interpretation of potentially frightening occurrences and used it as a source of her own help. She was able to see her son's naïve question and resolution as innocent and pure, giving her the strength to talk about and face the impending separation from Mel. They pulled together during those days, with Mel continuing to share his vision, giving a peace and release Donna had not known.

Mel came from the Jewish tradition, and Donna told me that her background had been Christian. She expressed that what was happening superseded any of their past beliefs. Once again, I felt privileged to be in their company. My gratitude at what was being offered made me feel ashamed at my earlier thoughts of disappointment in not leaving work early that day, and at the time I had wasted enumerating reasons I ought to feel resentful of a last-minute assigned visit.

Mel died shortly after this visit. I have thought often of Donna and Mel, of their palpable love that wasn't overt or mushy, but rather one of the purest expressions I have observed. I thought of a nine-year-old boy's "natural knowing" not to be fearful of the circle of life, which has to include death. I thought of Mel actually experiencing something that was merely a spark of light in my belief system. I thought often of this work that I was doing, and how it makes me feel connected to the universe in a substantial way. I thought about my purpose.

About a month later, I attended a presentation that included a discussion about gratitude, and its possible relation with the ideas of prosperity and abundance. It made some loose references to the idea of tithing, a church-related practice of giving money about which I knew little. I recall hearing that a tithe doesn't need to be exclusively associated with a church or religious affiliation; tithing can be broadened to include any source that spiritually nurtures. I considered this along with the many thoughts of my experiences with Donna and Mel.

It was just before Christmas, and I wrote a letter to Donna and enclosed a check. I described the powerful gifts that I felt I had received from our meetings. I asked her permission to share Mel's story with others who might be receptive, to give comfort. I offered an explanation for the check in terms of having been fed spiritually by her sharing with me Mel's journey. Finally, I asked for anonymity with regard to the funds I enclosed, as I had no idea whether this breached the bounds of professionalism in the view of anyone who had no awareness of the above disclosure. I expected no reply other than the endorsement on the check's reverse side; that would be enough.

Early in January, I received a letter from Donna. The following is part of it:

Dear Pato,

Thank you for your beautiful letter. I can honestly say that I have never received such a lovely letter. It touched me so much I really don't have the words to tell you.

Mel was a wonderful man and I know he

would be so pleased to have provided some peace of mind (and of soul!) to someone. He remembered your visits and spoke of you. We both appreciated your love and concern, caring ways. I read your letter to Mel. I like to think he hears me...

Anyway, your words made me have a bit more faith in life and people. It was so generous of you to send a check! I wanted you to know that I wanted the love in that check to continue making its way through the world. So, the boys and I took the check and went grocery shopping. We donated all the food to a local food pantry. My children learned how good giving feels and I could feel Mel all around us. Thank you, Pato, for such an elastic gift.

I'm so pleased that you wrote. I've wanted to tell you that you gave me strength. You treated me like a person at a time when I wanted to be a robot. You helped me realize even Mel's leaving was something to taste and savor and that he was still there to teach me something. And of course, as we both know, there was so much to be learned! Mel would be very happy to know that he was easing someone's pain—please keep sharing Mel with the world; it'll keep him alive for me...

Love, Donna

In an oral presentation, Dr. Bernie Siegel makes reference to "that wonderful gift we all get when the love is shared." Dr. Siegel continues, and in speaking of one of his Exceptional Cancer Patients, begins, "Because of the love he left…"

Mel and his wife, Donna, and her sons are all exceptional. They helped to facilitate my purpose: to give of myself so that others feel healed. And in so doing I, too, am healed because of the love. Thank you all for such an elastic gift.

First Baby

~

Kathy Ingallinera, RN

A DIAGNOSIS OF AIDS in the mid-1990s usually meant the patient was a young, gay male. Yolanda fit into only one of those categories. She was a young, straight female who was admitted with AIDS-related pneumonia to the medical intensive care unit where I worked.

Yolanda, age 19, lived in subsidized housing in a large inner-city project with her mom and several siblings. Like many teens, she hung out with her friends and had casual, unprotected sex with several different partners. If you had asked these kids about HIV, I'm sure you would have heard, "We don't have to worry about that 'round here. Ain't none of us gay."

Two years before her admission to the ICU, Yolanda went to a local clinic for a sports physical. After her doctor took Yolanda's history, she ordered testing for sexually transmitted diseases and was not surprised to get back a positive test for chlamydia. When the doctor called her to come back in for antibiotics, she talked with Yolanda about having some other STD tests done and also about the importance of using condoms. Yolanda reluctantly agreed to have blood drawn for HIV and syphilis.

Two weeks later, Yolanda listened to her phone messages when she got home from school. The first one said, "This is a message for Yolanda. This is Dr. Heddon's office. Please call as soon as possible." She hit DELETE and went to hang out with her friends.

A message appeared on the answering machine a week later. "Yolanda, this is Dr. Heddon. Please give me a call. It's urgent." DELETE.

A certified letter came in the mail several weeks later with the return address of Dr. Heddon's clinic. Yolanda's mom, Roberta, signed for it and gave it to her when she came home.

"What's this?" she said as she handed the letter to Yolanda.

"How should I know? I have to open it to know what it says," Yolanda said, angrily ripping the envelope open.

"Oh my God!" Yolanda gasped and held the paper to her chest. "I have AIDS!"

At Roberta's insistence, Yolanda made an appointment with Dr. Heddon, who told her she did not have AIDS but was HIV-positive and referred her to an infectious disease specialist at the Medical College of Virginia Hospital, where I worked. She was started on AZT and did well for a while. Unfortunately, she ended up in the emergency room almost two years after her diagnosis with a cough, fever, and shortness of breath. She was in respiratory distress, so she was intubated, placed on a ventilator, and admitted to the ICU, where I met her and Roberta.

It was discovered on admission lab work that Yolanda was pregnant. An ultrasound showed her to be around 20 weeks pregnant. When Yolanda was able to write notes, she communicated that she had known she was pregnant for the past four months, but had hidden it from her mom. She had been getting prenatal care through her HIV clinic.

Yolanda was ecstatic about the baby and interested in its development. Every four hours, we checked for fetal heart tones with a Doppler, documenting them on Yolanda's vital-sign sheet. She would lie in bed with a grin as we moved the Doppler back and forth through the gel across her slippery stomach until we heard the rapid pulse of the baby. When she heard the heartbeat, too, her face would break into a huge smile.

Yolanda's pretty face brightened even more with that smile. Her mocha-brown skin was framed by long, plaited dark-chocolate hair. She was short but sturdily built, and had been playing guard on her school basketball team before she got sick.

We kept close track of Yolanda's vital signs and asked her about fetal movement several times a day. Yolanda followed the baby's condition along with us, and we kept a picture of the ultrasound image on the corkboard on the wall where she could see it constantly.

One day melted into another in the hot Virginia summer. Yolanda had visitors every day, sometimes her oldest brother or a few girlfriends or her frail grandmother, who seemed confused by the whole scenario. Roberta visited every day, bringing small stuffed animals, fruity-smelling lotion, or helium balloons with cheery "Get Well" messages.

Roberta filled the room with her presence. Tall, big-boned, and dark-skinned, she dressed in African-inspired clothing, colorful and gauzy.

After Yolanda had been in the ICU for more than a week, a care conference was held. All of the primary nurses, her intern and resident doctors, the infectious disease team, an obstetrics-gynecology doctor, and the chief of the pulmonary team met with Yolanda and her mom to discuss her progress and plan of care.

It was decided that a tracheostomy would be performed to further assist her breathing. Despite antibiotics, tube feedings, and other supportive care, Yolanda's pneumonia was stubborn. Although she was slowly improving, she was going to be on the ventilator for at least another week.

Yolanda was in good spirits and getting out of bed every day. The baby was growing normally. Once Yolanda was off the ventilator, another ultrasound would be done to further assess the baby's growth and development. Yolanda smiled and wrote: "I am living for this baby!"

In the mid-1990s, the Food and Drug Administration had just approved the use of AZT in pregnant women to help reduce transmission of HIV to the child. We were hopeful that this baby might end up being HIV-negative, because Yolanda had remained on her AZT throughout her pregnancy.

The next morning I was in charge and taking care of one of my patients when Martha, the nurse who had been caring for Yolanda, called me aside, white-faced. "I can't hear fetal heart tones," she said in a scared hush. I quickly finished what I was doing and went with her to Yolanda's bedside.

Yolanda stared up at me, her eyes sad and wide. Her hair lay plaited in flat braids that surrounded her face. Tears rolled down her cheeks and soaked into the neckline of her blue hospital gown. I picked up the Doppler wand and searched without success for sounds of her baby's heartbeat.

"I'm sorry, Yolanda. I can't hear him either. Let me call your doctor and get an ultrasound ordered. Don't give up hope yet; maybe we just couldn't find him in there." I squeezed her hand and went to page her intern and her mom.

A portable ultrasound machine was rolled up to Yolanda's bedside and the colorful striped curtain was pulled around her bed to provide some privacy. Roberta had come as soon as we called, and now she sat beside the bed, holding Yolanda's hand.

When the procedure was complete, the radiology

technician called the radiologist, who looked at the films. He then called the obstetrician, who came and read the radiologist's notes and reviewed the film. Then he went behind the curtain with Yolanda's intern and nurse to give them the news. The baby, a girl, was dead.

The nurse and doctors came out ten minutes later and left Roberta and Yolanda behind the pulled curtain. Martha walked toward the central nurses' station and motioned for me to follow.

"I can't believe this," Martha started. "She wants to be taken off the ventilator to die. She pointed to that note hanging at the foot of her bed—'I am living for this baby'—and made a slashing motion across her throat." There were tears in her eyes.

"How is Roberta doing?" I asked.

"She was crying, trying to talk Yolanda out of it. Yolanda just kept shaking her head *No*."

Martha wiped her eyes and looked up as Roberta ducked out from behind the curtain.

I went to Roberta to hug her. "Not now, girl. I got to go call my pastor," Roberta said. She gave me a quick hug back and started out the door. "I'll be back."

I went to Yolanda's bed. She was on her side, facing away from the unit, looking out the window across an alley to another brick building. I sat by her. Tears were streaming down her face, dripping onto the bed, her shoulders shaking. I laid one hand on her arm and stroked her hair with my other.

"I'm so sorry, Yolanda. What can I do?" I squeezed

her hand. She shook her head: *No*. Then she turned suddenly onto her back and motioned for the clipboard and pencil. She wrote: "Call my doctor. Call my mom. I want to be with my baby." She sobbed.

"Your mom will be back in a few minutes. She went to call her pastor. Your doctor is right over there." I pointed to the counter at the nurses' station, where her intern sat talking on the phone while jotting some notes. "I'll tell him you want to see him as soon as he is done." She nodded and turned away.

I walked over and heard the intern say, "Okay. Thanks, Dr. Singh, I'll call you tomorrow." He hung up and turned to me. "Just got off the phone with psych. They'll come and evaluate her competency tomorrow." He pointed toward Yolanda as he continued: "We've got to wait 48 hours after the death of the baby before they'll consider taking her off of the ventilator. We have to give her time to really think about it. I mean, she can recover from her pneumonia and try to have another baby if she wants…" He looked at me. "I sure don't want her to die, but she seems pretty set. She'll probably still feel the same in a few days. By the way, she wants to talk to you, so you can go break the news to her."

Roberta came up to the unit with her pastor. Yolanda was asleep by then, so Roberta sat talking quietly with him. She stepped out to speak with me when she saw me peek around the curtain.

"Dr. Allen told me what the psychiatrist said and I am happy for that extra time. We will be praying, both here and at our church, for her to change her mind." She gave me a weak smile.

"Let me know if I can do anything. I don't pray much, but I sure will be thinking of you both."

"Are you working tomorrow?" Roberta asked.

"I'll be back in the morning. Give Yolanda a good-night hug for me. I have got to get home on time tonight. Friends are having a cookout and my husband is waiting there for me…"

"Go on, girl. We'll be here tomorrow. Have a good time." Roberta gathered me into a motherly hug, releasing me with a playful shove.

I had a hard time enjoying the cookout, my mind wandering back to Yolanda and her baby. I didn't envy Yolanda or her mom, but I understood their positions. It was a real ethical dilemma. I tried to put them out of my mind long enough to enjoy a cold beer, a burger, and some coleslaw. I succeeded…mostly.

The next day passed quietly. A kind, soft-spoken psychiatrist spent an hour talking with Yolanda. It was agreed at the outset of the meeting that no definite plans would be carried out that day. Time was spent making sure that Yolanda understood all of her options and that her doctors understood Yolanda's beliefs and hopes. At the end of the meeting Yolanda remained firm on her plan. She wanted to stop treatment, have the ventilator and breathing tube removed, and receive some sedation to keep her comfortable. If she survived, she would be moved from the ICU to a bed on a medical floor. If not, she would be with her baby.

The rest of the day went on as normally as possible. Yolanda got out of bed, sat in her chair to watch TV, received tube feedings and antibiotics, and visited with her family, friends, and pastor. She seemed at peace, waiting patiently for her plan to be carried out.

I would not be working the next day, so I stopped by Yolanda's bed to say good-bye to her and Roberta. I knew this was going to be difficult but I had to do it. If not, I would regret it forever.

Sticking my head around the curtain, I said, "Hey, you guys. I'm heading home and won't be in tomorrow. I wanted to stop and say good-bye."

I pulled a chair up next to the bed and took Yolanda's hand in mine. "How are you doing, honey?"

She picked up her clipboard and wrote: "I'm doing okay. Thank you for everything."

"You're welcome. Thank you, too."

"For what?" she wrote.

"For letting me take care of you, for teaching me what's important. You're a strong young woman, sticking to what you believe, and I admire that." I swiped my eyes with the side of my hand.

Roberta got up from her chair and sat on the edge of the bed. "Thanks for your help, Kathy."

"You've been a great support for her, Roberta. You've been here every day and that means a lot to Yolanda and also to the nurses. It's great to have a caring family member to talk with." I leaned over and hugged Roberta, squeezing her hard before I let go.

I sat looking at Yolanda. We were both crying and trying to smile, which made us cry all the more. "I won't forget you, Yolanda. I hope things go well tomorrow and you get what you want." I choked out, "Give that baby a hug and a kiss for me when you see her," as I leaned over and held her in my arms for a few minutes, then stood up, planted a big kiss on her forehead, and left.

The next evening I had a class at the School of Nursing, so I stopped by the unit to see how the day had gone. Martha had been her nurse that day, and told me tearfully that everything had gone according to Yolanda's plan.

The endotracheal tube was removed in the morning with Roberta and Pastor Whiting at the bedside. Yolanda's family came and visited for a while, then Yolanda requested some medication to help her relax so she could sleep. Even though her pneumonia had improved some, the removal of the breathing tube meant she had to do all the work of breathing on her own now, and she was tired.

The plan was to transfer her out of the ICU, but Yolanda passed away peacefully before Martha could call and give the report to the accepting nurse on the floor. Many of the ICU nurses thought Yolanda had given up her will to live, and that may be. I think she just wanted to see that baby badly enough that she simply slipped away. Either way, she got her wish.

Caring for Mr. B

~

Nkiru Okammor

I LIKE TO CONFRONT my fears. One of my fears working as a nurse is witnessing death and dying. In fall 2007, on one of my regularly scheduled 12-hour days, I had to face that fear.

Mr. B was a relatively healthy retired police officer, but he had a medical history of diabetes. Two years earlier, he was in a motor vehicle accident and never fully recovered. After acute care and rehab, he was transferred to a rehab nursing home for close monitoring. He then was transferred back to University of Michigan's health system because of some medical issues.

Mr. B had been placed on comfort care. Other nurses who took care of him reported that he was awake and even combative at times during the prior week. However, his health had deteriorated during the weekend. He started having more mental status changes and physiological issues.

This was the first time I had taken care of Mr. B, and during my initial assessment, he did not respond to any stimuli and was not blinking his eyes—he only had a blank stare. His pulmonary system took a turn for the worse and he began trying to compensate by using accessory muscles, with respirations in the upper 30s and 40s and on six liters nasal cannula. He also had tremors and restlessness at the beginning of the shift. After 8 AM, I gave him his morphine and Ativan IV, which were scheduled for every four hours and six hours, respectively.

I was angry about the frequency of the morphine and Ativan order, so I paged the doctor immediately to advocate for a change. The MD mentioned that the orders were written that way because Mr. B might be going to hospice. I estimated that Mr. B's condition had deteriorated to the extent that he might not survive the next 24 hours.

Because of my concern and the conversation I had with the MD, the morphine order was changed from every four hours to every two hours and the Ativan order from every six hours to every four hours. However, I still was not satisfied because the patient did not look comfortable even with the order change. When I saw the hospice team evaluating Mr. B, I approached them and expressed my concern about his p.r.n. medications. They heard the anger and concern in my voice and agreed with me; they understood my position, and so further changes were made. Although the morphine drip that I had suggested was not ordered, the morphine IV was finally changed to every hour and the Ativan IV to every two hours. I hoped that this would make Mr. B more comfortable.

While I was working on increasing the frequency of the p.r.n medications or initiating a morphine drip, I also became the family's advocate. Mr. B's wife, who happened to be a nursing administrator at the hospital, requested that a sitter stay temporarily with Mr. B. I asked the charge nurse to request a trained volunteer to stay at his bedside. In the meantime, I asked a tech to sit with the patient. As luck would have it, and to my surprise, a sitter was sent around 9 AM.

Once the sitter was in place, my next goal was to move Mr. B and his family to a private room for their grieving process. Because Mr. B's wife was a hospital employee, many people were coming in to visit him, causing a human traffic jam because he was in a semiprivate room. I asked the charge nurse at the beginning of the shift to secure the next private room for Mr. B. It seemed as though the plan would work, because a patient in a nearby private room had recently been discharged. I was patiently waiting for this room to be cleaned so that we could do the transfer when, to my surprise, I noticed that a new patient was slotted for this very room. I immediately consulted with the charge nurse to call the admitting office and cancel or transfer the new patient to a different room. I fought for Mr. B, and he and his family were transferred to this empty room as soon as the admission issue was resolved.

As hours went by, Mr. B was still in the process of dying, but he was much more comfortable. I administered the IV morphine, Ativan, and an eye drop almost every hour. I also spent a lot of time listening to his wife and other family members.

Mr. B passed away overnight. I think that might have been his way of thanking me for making him a little more comfortable. Perhaps in some way, he knew how I fear the dead and waited so as to not pass away during my shift.

Although Mr. B's death was sad, I felt good about accomplishing all of the nursing goals that I had set for him and his family. By helping to alleviate some of his pain and acting as the family's advocate, I felt reassured about the value of my role as a nurse.

An End to the Madness

∼

Emily McGee, RN

WE EACH DEAL with death in a different way. As nurses we are expected to remain strong, rarely discussing how we are affected emotionally by our jobs.

I opened my email a few weeks ago and cringed: yet another requirement to be fulfilled in the next three weeks for our accreditation, eight hours of clinical to be shoehorned into an already insane schedule. Opening day of trauma season had come and gone, so the slow winter shifts were officially over.

Cardiology has always been a weak area for me. I used to look at Chris (one of my fellow students and partners in crime) during my grad school days and laugh as he made a box with his hands over his heart saying, "This is all I care about, Emily. You can have the rest." His great interest was cardiology—about which I would passionately express my distaste.

Fast-forward to a conversation with Ben, who works in a cardiothoracic intensive care unit. He, too, loves everything about cardiology; he has an amazing passion for it. So as the stars aligned, I received permission to spend a shift with him.

Because I have no credentials at his institution, I was looking forward to 12 hours of being the newbie. You remember those days: no license to do anything other than follow an experienced nurse around with awe in your eyes. Strange to be back in that mindset knowing what I now know.

Late in the day, we recovered a double bypass patient, but this story isn't about Swan-Ganz catheters, cardiac parameters, or vasoactive drips. This is about another patient: one who gave much more to me than I to him, as only our patients can do.

David's spinal surgery went well. Although his extensive cardiac history made it risky, the surgeon deemed him well enough for the operating room, his young chronological age, I'm sure, being part of the decision-making process. His physiological age seemed much greater. HIV had done a number on him, as had his multiple previous myocardial infarctions.

Just prior to discharge, the patient suffered "the big one": a heart attack that landed him in the CT-ICU, assigned to Ben, and by default, to me. His DNR/DNI (do not resuscitate/do not intubate order) was a source of early discussion.

David became an exercise in clinical medicine versus patient care.

I have known Ben for quite some time in a U.S. Army capacity and as a friend. Caring for David with him opened my eyes to a side of Ben that could have taken years for me to see otherwise.

The intern shed her lab coat and took an inordinate amount of time to gather her supplies. Somehow the physicians convinced David to have an arterial line inserted. To Ben and me, it was obvious that this was something he didn't want. David knew his days were numbered and was at peace with this fact. They explained in depth how the muscle of his heart was not going to continue working well. At best he would have debilitating congestive heart failure for the remainder of his life, and they needed the a-line to get an accurate measure of his blood pressure and, therefore, be able to treat him.

David's partner was at his side, doting on him. They discussed what he should do, and David reluctantly agreed to the a-line. He knew that it was a temporary measure only, to help with temporary treatment. While the obviously nervous resident went about setting up her sterile field, Ben and I intermittently spent time at David's bedside with wet cloths for his forehead and conversation to distract him from the looming procedure. Ben's easy manner, quick smile, and confidence permeated the room, putting David at ease.

Earlier that day, Ben had turned the corner with a grin from ear to ear. "Emily, you know how long David and his partner have been together?"

I shook my head, trying not to smile at the almost mischievous grin plastered on his face.

"Twenty-nine years!"

As we were all packed in David's room, it was inevitable that Ben ask where David met his partner.

David's mother had warned us earlier about the extent of David's wicked sense of humor. We were given brief peeks at it when he mustered enough energy for a zinger, cracking us up throughout the day.

David did not hesitate in responding to Ben's inquiry. "I met him in the orgy room of the Adonis Club. He was the only one I ever had breakfast with." His grin at the memory and joy at the expected reaction we gave him was something I will never forget. David lived life his own way, and it showed even when he was lying ill in an ICU bed.

As the resident proceeded to attempt small talk, thinking it was hiding her nervousness at the procedure, Ben and I exchanged looks over the bed. This was going to be ugly. Although we kept an eye on the monitor, watching David's low pressure measured by the BP cuff, we instead focused on his pale face, on his forehead beading with sweat. Ben brought more wet cloths. I held David's hand.

Throughout my training I have done those difficult procedures, and been nervous as I felt all eyes on me. I also knew when to quit. I knew when to actually look at my patient and give him permission to say no. The inside of my cheek and lip were almost bloody as I kept bit-ing them to keep me from saying something that was not my place to say. I could see it in Ben's eyes as well. We exchanged a glance and I quietly walked out. Ben slid up to David and took my place.

There was an order to make David NPO (nothing by mouth) and neither the intern, the resident, nor the chief resident knew why ("Guess it was just in case Cardiology wanted to do a procedure"). They didn't even question it, but instead just wrote it. There was no way on earth a cardiologist was going to touch David. Where was the critical thinking needed to do what was right for David?

At some point I reentered the room, after giving Ben an exasperated look when no one could see me but him.

The resident decided he was going to take over stabbing David's radial artery. After tucking his tie into his dress shirt, he put on sterile gloves that were way too large.

On his way to the clean utility room, he stated, "Well, guess I am a 7.5, not an 8!"

Before any of us could blink, David piped up, "Well, I wouldn't go around bragging about that!"

Ben and I almost lost it, we were laughing so hard.

After coming back and going through another three catheters unsuccessfully, the resident stopped to discuss what to do next with the chief resident, who at some point had appeared in the room. While the residents were discussing the difficulty of getting the catheter placed, Ben and I quietly told David it was okay to take a break and by giving him that permission, enabled him to put an end to the madness.

After clarifying the NPO orders and cleaning up the mess the residents left, we spent the remainder of our time with David making him as comfortable as possible. I stood to the side while David's mother and sisters thanked Ben for everything he had done, his mother close to tears. She had recently lost not only her husband but her brother, too, and now was on the verge of losing her son.

Without stopping to think, Ben reflexively stepped forward and pulled this small woman into a protective, caring embrace, which she unhesitatingly and gratefully accepted.

Wicked Codes

∽

Karen Klein, RN, BSN, CEN

It was about four o'clock in the morning toward the end of a busy Saturday night shift when the notification came that a gunshot victim was on the way in to the New York City emergency room where I worked. The weary crew I was working with suddenly sprang to action, roused by the prospect of saving a life.

When the patient arrived, I faded into the background and assisted the others in the trauma team. I was new to ER nursing, having started working there only a few months earlier and still not fully confident in my skills.

The bullet had entered this man's left upper chest. He was unconscious and in cardiac arrest. I watched as the trauma team worked on the patient, including doing chest compressions to keep his blood flowing, intubating and ambuing to breathe for him, applying monitor leads, and putting in large-bore IVs. At one point, the doctor inserted a chest tube to see if there was bleeding in the chest. The nurse had set up for the tube and once it was in, she connected it to the suction canister, which has the capacity to hold a liter and a half of fluid. I remember watching the canister fill up immediately, as if the blood were being poured in from a pitcher. I didn't have very much trauma nursing experience, but that seemed like a lot of blood to lose. My thought was confirmed when one of the nurses grunted, "Uh oh," and then hooked the tube up to a second suction canister, which filled with another half liter of blood.

I didn't know the progression of a trauma, but the nurse clearly did.

"Ya gonna crack the chest, doc?" she inquired as she reached for the equipment tray to do just that.

"Yup," the doctor replied.

I had never before witnessed what they called "cracking the chest." Basically, this means making a large incision in the left side between the ribs, separating the ribs with retractors, and reaching in the chest with a gloved hand to feel whether the heart still had any blood in it. It's a last-ditch effort to determine the patient's viability and, if the heart does have blood, to give internal cardiac massage or even shock the heart directly in order to save the patient.

I watched as the incision was made, the retractors were placed and pulled back, and the doctor reached into the man's open chest. It was, admittedly, somewhat brutal to behold.

"This heart is empty. He's got a hole in his left ventricle," the doctor stated. "It's done. Thank you, everybody."

Immediately, the entire trauma team walked out of the room, leaving only one nurse, the ER doctor, and myself with the newly deceased patient.

"That's it?" I questioned. Was there nothing more to be tried?

The doctor turned to me and said, "Put on some gloves."

He turned the man on his side. Just to the right of his left scapula (wing bone) was the clearly outlined lump of a bullet, its tip visible under the skin.

"That's where the bullet stopped," the doctor remarked. "Just as I thought. It went right through his left ventricle. Wanna feel the hole?" he asked.

Being new and eager to learn, I did. I put on a long glove that went nearly to my elbow and reached into the patient's chest. I felt the intact heart, placing my whole hand around it at first, holding it in my hand. Then I felt around the back of it, where there was a small hole just big enough for me to poke my index finger through.

"Wow!" I exclaimed, "I thought the hole would be larger. It doesn't feel very big."

"It doesn't need to be very big. When it's in the main pumping chamber of your heart, you bleed out in seconds," he responded.

I held the heart in my hand once more. It was almost surreal. I remember thinking this job was not like any other. In how many jobs can you literally hold a person's heart in your hand?

As it turned out, the deceased was a Japanese citizen who was in New York on business for a few weeks. His fiancée had flown in that weekend to spend a week with him and tour the city. They were going back to his hotel after a night out on the town when someone pulled a gun and demanded his wallet, which he would not give up. For that he was shot.

The fiancée spoke no English, and it wasn't until nearly six AM that we were able to grab a Japanese student, who happened to be walking by the hospital on his way to school, to translate and tell her that her fiancé was dead. Understandably, she became so hysterical that she, too, became a patient: We had to give her valium. I felt so bad for her. I couldn't imagine going to a foreign country to visit with my fiancé and seeing him get shot and killed. I have always felt that this poor woman probably left New York with no desire to ever return. I would imagine that for her, the mere mention of New York City will forever bring pangs of grief in remembrance of that one long dark, dreadful life-altering night.

For me, it was my first "wicked code." Unfortunately, it wouldn't be my last.

On another night shift in another hospital quite a few years later, our ER received a 19-year-old patient with a stab wound to the chest. He was unconscious, with a very rapid heart rate and virtually no blood pressure. The trauma surgeon cracked the chest, reached in, and felt around.

"The heart has blood," he told us, and then he asked for a large hemostat, a metal clamp used to compress a bleeding vessel.

"I've got the aorta in my hand. There's a nick in it. I want to cross clamp it, then we'll take him to the OR for repair," he informed the team. "Does he have any pupillary reaction?"

Because I happened to be standing at the head of the stretcher, I took the otoscope light to check the patient's pupillary response. I expected to find none, because the medics had said his pupils were fixed and dilated—a very bad sign. But when I shined the light in his left eye, I was stunned to find that it constricted.

Just as I started to declare my startling finding to the team, the patient suddenly sat up and began flailing his arms and legs...with the doctor's hand still in his chest!

Everybody in the room was stunned. The chances of a patient regaining consciousness after having his chest cracked are nearly nil—not to mention the mere sight of someone flailing about while a doctor has his hand inside the person's chest.

Naturally, the doctor was also taken aback, and he lost his grip on the aorta. He was never able to cross clamp with the hemostat. Instead the patient was rushed up to the operating room directly. I found out later that the patient died.

Later, we all discussed this bizarre incident and came to the conclusion that enough blood must have gone up to the patient's brain when the doctor was manually clamping the aorta to cause the patient to have a moment of semi-consciousness. I remember thinking that this patient's last act in life was to freak out a room full of medical practitioners. A truly wicked code if ever there was one.

One day at another ER, we coded a woman for more than an hour, so sure were we that we could bring her back. After all, she was only 52 years old, and her sudden heart attack seemed to have come out of nowhere. Bystanders at the scene did immediate CPR, and the medics were there within five minutes to administer advanced cardiac life support. According to the medics, her family said she had never been sick before. She had no medical history whatsoever, until this.

We worked as hard and fast as we could, but despite our doing everything medically possible, her heart simply refused to beat. Finally, the doctor called the code and asked for the time. We were all dejected.

I took the newly deceased patient off the monitor and the respiratory therapist disconnected the Ambu bag from the tube that was inserted into her lungs during the code. Suddenly she began to breathe. At first it seemed like just a sigh, but then she took one breath in and then exhaled. Then another inhalation, then an exhalation, then another, then another. The entire code team was standing around the stretcher, staring wide-eyed at her as she continued to "breathe." The doctor pulled the stethoscope out of his pocket and listened to her chest. "No, she has no heartbeat," he said. "That's it, folks. She's gone." Then he added, "But you should see the freaky look on all of your faces!"

I looked around at everyone—sure enough, all of their eyes were like saucers.

Later while some of us were discussing this wicked code, one senior nurse remarked that she had seen this phenomenon once before.

"How long did you say you coded her—an hour? Then it must have been muscle memory."

Someone questioned her as to what that meant and she explained.

"Sometimes if you code someone long enough and hyperventilate them for so long, the muscles of respiration just continue for a bit in an automatic-type way."

Muscle memory. It was a logical explanation. It made sense. But still, I'll never forget how strange it was to see a dead woman breathing. I filed it mentally under the term *wicked code*.

I once was asked how many people I had seen die in my more than 20 years of nursing. I had never really thought about it in terms of numbers. Was it a hundred? Two hundred? Five hundred? I couldn't really say. But some of those deaths stand out in my mind much more than others—especially the wicked codes.

There Are
No Coincidences

~

Patrice Piretti, RN-C

MY CAREER LED ME to a fulfilling position in a Long Island community health center providing primary nursing care to the uninsured and the underinsured. The fall of 2002 marked a season of reflection and personal growth, because my life was touched by a spirited young woman with an Irish brogue. Katie was referred to the health center by her breast surgeon because she had recently been diagnosed with breast cancer.

I remember so clearly the green-eyed beauty with a matching bandana covering what were once her strawberry curls. When I saw her, I wondered if she was a cancer patient.

The day before, I had also sat in the waiting room of a breast center filled with anxiety and apprehension. Earlier that week, I had found a lump during a breast self-exam. I recall the terror and distinct chill as I sat in a circular formation with other women dressed in paper gowns anxiously awaiting medical evaluation. The newcomers like me nervously tapped their feet or flipped through magazine pages. Women began to engage in conversation, which proved to be therapeutic. They verbalized their experiences and provided reassurance as well as support. I sat in this circular formation witness to the circle of hope.

The winter was uneventful for both Katie and me. She continued her treatment and I was carefully monitored by a breast surgeon. I looked forward to her monthly visits, because she would warm up the unit with her smile and positive attitude. At the end of each visit, I would be the recipient of a gentle embrace and words of Irish wisdom.

Spring 2003 had arrived, and Katie and I were relieved that the winter had come to an end. We both enjoyed the outdoors and experienced comfort from the ocean. The McCormack family reunion was to be held at my house that summer. Katie eagerly requested an update of the upcoming event at each office visit. The portrait of Grandma and Grandpa McCormack and their 12 children was proudly displayed in my living room that summer. Katie and I became hysterical when we discussed the family pencil-thin lips and long arms (physical characteristics we both shared). The nursing station was filled with laughter when we discussed the uniqueness of Irish wakes and funerals. We shared stories of our heritage, which elicited both sadness and joy. This special woman spoke about her long journey to America and the fulfillment of a childhood dream.

Katie's presence that summer connected me to the spirit of my great-great-grandmother. More than a century ago, an equally tenacious, spirited, and brave woman journeyed to America with her family in hopes of improving the quality of their lives. If one thing had been different in the life of Grandma McCormack, I might not be where I am today. I thanked Katie for awakening the spirit of my Irish heritage. Each event of my life, including the friendship with Katie, has contributed a rich thread to my personal tapestry, and for this I am grateful.

During fall 2003, Katie had become ill with various infections, which required frequent visits to the center. On Mondays, I would diligently check the appointment system to see if she had an upcoming visit. During each encounter she displayed courage and hope.

By the New Year, Katie had been admitted to the hospital several times. Her visits to the center had become less frequent, and I missed her company. On a Friday during the second week of March, I returned from lunch and heard the pleasant voice of my friend. As she exited the exam room, she was being held by her dedicated mother-in-law. As I gazed into Katie's eyes, I felt that something had changed, because the communication was incongruous. Her words were hopeful and courageous, but her eyes were saying good-bye. My special friend left the building and I cried inconsolably.

I returned to work on Monday and was informed that my precious friend had died on Sunday. A colleague held me tightly in her arms and said she was very sorry for my loss. This empathic nurse gently reminded me that Katie was free from pain and that I would always carry her spirit in my heart.

I sadly waved a final good-bye to Katie. Her casket, draped in green linen with a picture of St. Patrick, was gently placed in the hearse. I recall proudly thinking, "Homeward bound, Katie. Destination: Ireland. Date of departure: March seventeenth, St. Patrick's Day." There are no coincidences, only lessons to be learned.

I have since left my position at the health center and am currently working as a supervisor in my community hospital. The unique experience with Katie occurred because we both were fully present in the moment. This level of caring was influenced by our individual journeys and our respect for each other's human spirit. This mutual respect created an environment of trust, which strengthened our relationship and contributed to the healing process.

Every day I am privileged to witness caring nurses valuing the uniqueness of patients, families, and each other. I pledge to do the same with grace and dignity and will continue to provide an environment that fosters spiritual growth and trust. My continued growth will be determined by my ability to provide self-care and nurture my spiritual well-being.

While I was writing this story, a nurse entered the nursing office and said, "Happy St. Patrick's Day, Patrice." I didn't realize that the day was March 17, 2008. There are no coincidences—only lessons to be learned.

Defining Moments

~

Lisa Affatato, RN-BC

It has been said in nursing that every nurse has a defining moment. I had been a nurse for only about eight months when my moment began.

I remember walking into this patient's room for the first time. I was a little wary, because he seemed a little demanding and rough around the edges. He had a tracheotomy, which made him difficult to understand at times. When I went to give him his meds that morning, he abruptly told me he needed ice water to swallow the pills. I was on the next day as well, and this time I did not forget the ice water!

Slowly, we built a trust together. I seemed to understand him without his speaking. I knew just how to fluff and position the pillows, and easily lifted him out of the bed and into the chair. He trusted my "alley-oop" maneuver. We developed a routine that worked.

Rizz spent many months in the hospital, fighting hard every day—for himself and for his family. I spent 40 hours a week with him; I was as much a constant in his life as he was in mine. We talked about many things. I remember talking to him about a medication the doctors wanted him to take to ease his anxiety, which he was adamant about not taking. I explained how it would help him; he listened, knowing I was being truthful, and then came to rely on that medication. We had trust.

He was getting sicker and sicker, coming up on a year in the hospital. He was going to dialysis five times a week and going off our floor only for brief visits to the critical care unit. He always came back to us. In fact, the doctors would write orders to transfer him, but he always came back to my district.

I suppose I wasn't aware of what an impact he had on me, or that I had on him, until the last month of his life. The biggest event for us was being able to take him outside for his birthday—what a joyous day that was! The sun was warm, his wife brought his dogs, which he hadn't seen in about a year, and his face just lit up. He also ate ravenously that day; we couldn't get the chocolate-covered strawberries in fast enough!

Rizz started to talk to me about being tired and not wanting to fight anymore. We had many heart-to-heart conversations. I offered support and encouragement where I could. I told him to talk to his family about his wishes, that they would support him, and that they loved him so much.

My one regret is that I told him I would help him write letters to his family members. Unfortunately, that never happened, but I think they said everything they needed to each other. He struggled with signing his do-not-resuscitate order but did manage to sign it, and he stopped dialysis. He had his own personal battles to overcome regarding stopping this; he was struggling with the idea that doing so was a form of committing suicide. We had some long talks about this, during which I listened and offered my advice where appropriate. He was able to meet with his priest to discuss these issues and make his decision.

I had the opportunity to take him outside one more time. The sun was very warm that day, and I remember watching him stare into the blue sky and the fluffy white clouds for what seemed like a very long while; he was very still and quiet. When we got back indoors, he held my hand for a moment and said he wanted to be alone for a few minutes. I knew then that he was ready. I came in again another day to try to take him outside—I had promised him pizza! Unfortunately, I couldn't get him to wake up enough, so I sat with him for awhile, holding his hand and talking with him. He squeezed my hand one last time before I left. I got the call the next morning that he had passed during the night.

At first I was angry. I thought for sure I would be there for him, but he knew better in the end. It is a strange thing to feel so close to someone who is not family and who, in the scheme of things, you've only known a short time. But we had a bond. I took care of him for almost a year and I was grieving his loss.

There is such a flood of unexpected emotions that you are unsure of how to handle. And, as the nurse, no one is saying to you "sorry for your loss."

I learned, though, that in this situation you do go through the stages of grieving. This man and his family affected my life and my career in ways I am sure I have yet to learn. I know that my first day back after his passing was a tough one. I did not want anyone to be in "his" room. Of course, there was someone—thank goodness it was a woman, so I wouldn't be reminded of him! I am thankful that in the first few weeks we had a high turnover on the floor. I was afraid to become close to someone again. However, that's not me. It will happen again, and I will not be afraid.

I was glad to be able to go to the wake for Rizz. It was wonderful to see what a full life he had. It is not often that nurses get to see the whole person. The experience has helped me define my role as a nurse who has the ability to make a difference in someone's living. I also see how important it is to make a difference in someone's dying.

Pearls

~

Sarah Burns, RN

Beth was a 57-year-old mother of three grown daughters and a wife to a very devoted man named Greg. Beth had contracted hepatitis from a blood transfusion and received a liver transplant six months before. Her recovery was complicated by kidney failure and a need for dialysis, an engorged spleen, osteomyelitis, and several tunneling wounds. Now she was in our intensive care unit for respiratory failure, infection, and continuous dialysis.

Taking care of Beth was a challenge. She had been off sedation for 48 hours and still wouldn't open her eyes to command, but she grimaced when we suctioned her and she lifted her hand a little bit. Her pupils were equal and reactive to light: no evidence of bleeding in her head. With her liver and kidney failure, it was difficult to tell whether she was capable of becoming any clearer mentally. The liver transplant team and our doctors had spoken with the family the day before; I knew that at the very least, they thought Beth's status should be changed to "do not resuscitate," meaning if her heart stopped, we would not restart it with CPR and drugs.

I got a report from the night nurse and went in the room. Greg was there, along with two of their daughters. He told me they had held a meeting. I adjusted the numbers on the dialysis machine, suctioned Beth's breathing tube, and then sat down with them. They went over what the doctors had told them the night before: that they'd made Beth a DNR and were considering withdrawing aggressive therapies.

One of the daughters was a nurse, and she was concerned that there might be one more thing we could do. "I know things don't look good," she said. "But I guess because she's moving her hand now, if she has a chance at all, I don't want to take it from her."

I told her I understood. Of course she wanted to give her mother every chance. It would almost be easier if Beth were bleeding in her head—no neurosurgeon would operate on someone so sick, as her brain would herniate and it would all be over. We reviewed Beth's long fight with cirrhosis, the liver transplant, and multiple infections. With each complication she had become weaker and lost some ground. Greg said he believed that this was more than she could recover from.

He cleared his throat and put his arm around his daughter. He told us that Beth was getting tired of hospitals and medications. Since the transplant, she had been at home for a total of 12 days. The rest of the time was spent in the hospital or at clinic visits. The daughter nodded. I explained that for a person who has three or more organ systems failing, the morbidity is extremely high. I reviewed Beth's body systems: Her spleen was engorged, necessitating platelet transfusions every 12 hours; her transplanted liver was not clearing waste products and making clotting factors the way it should; and her kidneys had shut down, making her dependent on dialysis to maintain her pH and clear her waste products and fluids. Then I described her wounds, which weren't healing because she wasn't absorbing the nutrition she needed. And she was still on a ventilator and a little medication to keep her blood pressure up. The family understood that even if Beth made it off the ventilator and out of the ICU, her rehab time would be months and months.

The daughters left to shower. I consolidated the IV pumps and got rid of some extra pillows and equipment. Greg sat down at the head of the bed and started talking about all the nice places he and Beth had traveled. "Remember when that family of raccoons visited our campsite?" he laughed. "You were the hero, leading them away with that corn."

I emptied the dialysis bag, drew some blood, and reduced the blood pressure medicine. Occasionally I would comment on part of the story and Greg would flesh it out for me. The rest of the time I left them alone to reminisce.

The doctors rounded and I relayed our conversation to them. They shared what they had learned from the family meeting the day before. They said hello to Greg, and we all agreed that they would return after rounds to talk to the family further. The daughters returned with some other family members. The hesitant daughter told me they had all talked. "I know she wouldn't want this. This isn't a meaningful life for her," she said.

The conversation turned quickly to the withdrawal process of dialysis and the ventilator. For 25 minutes I sat there and answered questions about what death would look like. "Will she die right away?" they asked me. I told them probably not. Often when people are on high amounts of blood pressure medicine and are then taken off them, they die quickly. But Beth required only a small amount of medicine to keep her blood pressure up. So how would she die? I explained that once we stopped dialysis, her blood wouldn't be continuously buffered, so the waste products would build up. Her pH was already low. It would get lower, the heart muscle would become irritable, and the blood pressure would drop. That would make the heart more irritable.

I explained that an irritable heart might beat too fast or too slowly but either way, in time, it would slow down and stop. They asked about Beth's breathing. I told them they could make a choice: If they chose to take the breathing tube out, her breathing might look more labored and it could be difficult to clear the secretions in the back of the throat. But some families want to see the patient pass away without any tubes or drains. Or they could leave the tube in and we would just lower the ventilator support. I assured them that we would be there with pain medications if they thought she was in any discomfort. The doctors returned and spoke with the family. They wrote orders according to the family's wish: Leave the breathing tube in, lower the ventilator support, and medicate for pain.

Finally all the decisions were made and the family left the room for a break. I returned Beth's blood to her and disconnected the dialysis machine, gave her a bath and some pain medicine, changed the sheets, and cleared off the counters. I rounded up three more chairs and a few more boxes of tissues and put them in the room.

When the family was ready, the respiratory therapist came in and lowered the ventilator settings. I turned off all the IV fluids and blood pressure medication. The family pulled their chairs up to the bed and they held Beth's hands. The minister from Beth's home church was in the room. Together the family prayed, told stories, and cried.

I left it up to them to tell me if they thought Beth needed pain medication. After awhile we decided together on a morphine drip. I brought them a bereavement food tray, made coffee, and answered questions. The EKG monitor was reading continuously, but I checked the blood pressure and oxygen saturation only every hour. I find that families can sometimes fixate on the numbers, so we turn the monitors off, but it's also nice to know how things are progressing. The blood pressure and oxygen saturation dropped slowly, and after awhile the heart rhythm changed. Finally, Beth's heart stopped.

The doctor came and pronounced death, and the respiratory therapist turned the ventilator off. The family was outside the room. I hugged each of the daughters and told them what I tell all the families: that I wish we could have done more, wish we had a magic wand, how sorry we are for their loss. I went back in the room and took the pearl earrings out of Beth's ears. I put them in a little bag. When I turned around, Greg was standing there. "Sarah," he said, putting his hand on my shoulder. "I just…" He stopped and took a deep breath. "You made Beth comfortable and we all thank you." I handed him the bag with the earrings and gave him a hug.

He's Coming

~

Mary DeLisle-Berry, RN

HER NAME WAS HELEN. She was a 72-year-old woman dying of chronic obstructive pulmonary disease (COPD). I was her hospice nurse. One thing I've always loved about doing hospice nursing is the opportunities I've had to really get to know people. It is probably appropriate to add "and provide good nursing care and support at the end of life." And I have done that; I have provided good nursing care to dying people. But that is a given for hospice nurses, I think. Good nurses provide good nursing care at every stage of life. In hospice, however, the boundaries that define giver and receiver often fog; it is not always so clear who's providing what for whom. I've always seen it as a dance, with no assigned steps; the only given rule I knew was that the patient always gets to lead.

During the time I had getting to know Helen, she invited me into her heart. She told me stories of her life, sharing memories and dreams with me. I was her hospice nurse for six months. In acute care settings, these kinds of conversations don't always take place. ER visits, hospital admissions for the administration of the latest life-saving drugs and treatments, and the focus on "fighting the good fight" is the focus there. But in hospice, once comfort needs are met, there is time to be spent reflecting on life, its purpose and meaning.

During one of my early conversations with Helen, we talked about what death meant to her. She told me she was a Christian woman and her Bible was a source of comfort and hope to her. Her ideas about death were grounded in her faith. Often she would share Scripture passages and inspirational stories she was reading with me when I visited her. One day she shared with me a recurring dream she was having. She kept dreaming of her father; he had died when she was very young. He had been a helicopter pilot.

She had a picture of him in his aviator uniform: a young man in his twenties. He was holding the hand of an adoring little five-year-old girl. Helen remembered that picture being taken. You'd think the years would have lessened her memories of him, but they had not. She remembered how much she loved him and how tender he was with her. In the dream she was having she said, "My father is there. He tells me not to be afraid. He says he will come for me, and take me home, when it is time to go." When she would awaken from this dream, Helen always felt so peaceful. She told me that as crazy as it might sound, she believed it. She believed that when it was her time to die, her father really would be there for her.

I went to a hospice conference recently in Dublin, Ireland. One of the speakers referred to an ancient Celtic practice at the time of dying. A specific role existed in which a healer was assigned to be an Anam Cara (the literal translation is "soul friend") to the dying person. The Anam Cara would help the dying person make the transition by being alongside that person through the process, attending to his or her physical, emotional, and spiritual needs. He said it was this practice that provided the early roots of our modern hospice movement. Well, I was Helen's soul friend. I ministered to her physical and emotional needs during my time as her nurse. And she took me into her world, telling me her stories and dreams. I never thought any of them were crazy. We'd made an agreement that I would remind her of that dream of her father when death was near. And I did.

Helen had the same physical deterioration process going on that I had seen in many people with COPD. Air hunger eventually narrowed her focus. Each breath became a mantra: breathing in, breathing out. The effort to breathe kept her ever present in its demand. The term for this—*air hunger*—is an interesting one, now that I reflect on it. During the months I was her hospice nurse, our conversations became shorter and shorter as she needed to conserve air more and more for breathing. It was difficult to watch her labor. My job at that point was to make sure she optimized her oxygen and that she did so as painlessly as possible. And I did, using all my hospice skills of symptom management. I often, however, found myself thinking about our earlier conversations about her dad and her belief that he would be there for her at the time of death. It seemed a long time ago that we had talked about such things. The smells and sounds and feel of death had me focusing on supporting Helen's physical needs, and her job was to breathe. And rest.

The night Helen died, I was the on-call nurse for hospice. It was about three AM and I was awakened from a deep sleep. A distinctive sound shook me into consciousness—a whirling, winded sound. I sat bolt up right abruptly—I swear this is true—awakened by the sound of a helicopter outside my window! Then the phone rang. In a daze, I picked up the receiver. It was the answering service for hospice. A woman's voice told me that Helen had just died. Incredulously, I said, "I know."

I've shared that story with many people. Some ask me if I had "seen the helicopter." Well, I didn't run to the window—I got up and answered the phone. Others ask if I think I was perhaps dreaming that I heard a helicopter. I don't know the answer to that for sure; I just know the sound of a whirlybird's wings woke me up. And when very shortly after I picked up the phone and heard that Helen had died, I felt completely at peace. Helen's death has taken me to places of reflection and wonder—places

I had never been before I met her. My inner world has grown because of it. Who, I ask myself, really was the giver? Who was the receiver in this time I spent with Helen? What a dance!

First Night

~

Cortney Davis, MA, RN-C, APRN

AFTER COMPLETING MY final year of nursing school, after taking my nursing boards and receiving the envelope that held my license—proof of my expertise—I became a real nurse in a real job, working the night shift in intensive care.

My nursing program had been a rigorous combination of clinical and academic work. By graduation, I'd run a floor, taken care of ventilator patients, started intravenous lines, passed meds, participated in codes, and, in general, was ready to hit the ground running. And so, after an eight-week heart-monitoring course, I found myself in charge of a seven-bed intensive care unit, the only registered nurse on the night shift. I had a nurse's aide to help me, a woman in her fifties with 30 years of experience, and I had the support of the night supervisor, who floated about from floor to floor, pushing the 3 AM snack cart, holder of the keys to the pharmacy and the morgue, and the one to call in case of an emergency. But despite the aide and the supervisor, in that small unit of desperately ill patients, the buck stopped with me.

On my first night as charge nurse, I walked in to find two patients with fresh myocardial infarctions, an elderly post-op, and four ventilator patients, one of them a ten-year-old girl who had been hit by a car and was dying.

Was I scared? I was terrified.

Everything was different back then. The intensive care beds, separated by glass half-walls and long curtains, fanned out around a central nurse's station, a long desk where seven monitors beeped and pinged, echoing the rhythms of the seven monitors at the patients' bedsides, an odd, syncopated song that never stopped. There was an absence of computers—and an absence of paperwork. An intake and output sheet hung by each patient's bedside; a nursing cardex held one page for each patient, and on that card was written a succinct nursing care plan and any important information about allergies, code status, and next of kin. Nurses' and doctors' notes were handwritten in the chart, available for all to read with a minimum of effort. And the change-of-shift report was given to the incoming nurses face-to-face, not taped or typed into a computer to be printed and passed along like a secret note. In other words, we had a lot less aggravation and a lot more time to spend with our patients.

And spend time with patients we did. In intensive care, there was no such thing as "rounds"—in our small unit, we were with our patients constantly. During the day, when most of the activity took place, there was a low patient-to-nurse ratio. Because we had no interns or residents, we nurses started and restarted IVs, placed or replaced nasogastric tubes, pushed curare to keep our ventilator patients sedated, and, because respiratory techs were not yet a common part of the team, we adjusted ventilator settings, ordered blood gasses, and then readjusted the vents to maintain doctor-ordered parameters.

Every patient was bathed once a day and "sponge bathed" in the evening, not with pre-packaged and pre-soaped disposable cloths but with real soap and water. Each immobile patient was turned regularly, some every 15 minutes. We gave back rubs three times a day, soaked and washed feet, got patients out of bed, and hounded them to take deep breaths, to cough, and to move.

Standing at the central nurses' station, I could see all my patients and, at the same time, watch their heart lines leap across the monitor screens in front of me. I could tell by a slight disturbance in the pattern when a patient was restless or having pain, and I knew that my duty was to go to and help that patient. Sometimes *help* meant sitting by the bedside and talking; other times it meant recognizing an impending disaster, calling the attending, and positioning the code cart right outside the curtain, out of the patient's sight.

I'd done all these things and more as a student, always with an experienced nurse somewhere nearby. Even so, that first night in charge, as I walked into that scene of agony and grief, I trembled as the evening charge nurse gave me report. I wasn't at all sure I would survive. I wasn't sure that I could help these patients survive and, more than that, I was afraid I might harm them. I'd never felt more alone.

"Little Jenny over there in cubicle three was hit by a car while riding her bike today," the evening nurse told me. "She has massive internal and neurological injuries, her blood pressure is dropping, they've got her paralyzed on a vent, and we can't control her heart rate. The docs expect her to die within the hour, and her dad won't leave her side."

I looked over at cubicle three. A thin girl, dark-haired, was barely visible in the bed. The respirator huffed beside her, and a spider web of tubes and catheters held her captive. Hovering over her was a man with tousled brown hair, glasses, and a baseball jacket. He looked as if he had run from his house without money or comb, without anything in the world but his daughter, who now was in what we rightly call the agony of death. The father held his daughter's hand, and I could hear him, his words muffled, as he pleaded with her to live. How could I, a new graduate — a well-trained one to be sure, but also one who didn't yet have the years of experience — handle all this?

The evening nurses and aides and ward clerk left, one by one, looking back over their shoulders at Jenny and her dad. As the automatic door whooshed closed, an eerie silence fell over the unit, interrupted only by the out-of-synch music of the respirators, each of them hissing its own tune, and the repeating voices of the seven monitors. The nurse's aide and I looked at each other.

"I'll do vital signs and make sure the IVs are okay," she said. She was probably just as frightened as I was, wondering if this new grad in her crisp white uniform was going to kill anyone that night.

I think maybe I did. I think I might have killed Jenny.

After all these years, I can't remember the exact sequence of events. In the middle of the night, when memory plays its tricks and dredges up the worst scenarios, the most awful implications, I think that I went first to Jenny's bedside before checking any other patients. I introduced myself to her father. I remember having tears in my eyes as I watched them, father and daughter. I recall reading the medication cardex, the order for the intravenous medication to be given if Jenny's pulse exceeded a certain rate. I remember her wildly racing heart, suddenly shooting up to well over 200 beats per minute, and I remember drawing up the medication and administering it. Then, shortly after this administration, I remember her dying.

It wasn't *then*, that night, that I wondered if I'd hastened Jenny's death. I didn't wonder this until years later, after I'd learned how human error and imperfect knowledge walk beside us nurses and doctors every minute of every shift. It wasn't until I'd had years of experience that I became familiar with how we caregivers can sometimes second-guess ourselves, especially when something suddenly goes wrong and we have to act instantly. That is when I thought of Jenny.

When I'm feeling sure of myself and my skills, I recall a different memory. She didn't die within minutes of receiving the medication, but hours later. I remember that the night supervisor, a friendly, gray-haired woman, came to the unit to sit in the waiting room with Jenny's mother, who couldn't bear to be with her dying child. I remember Jenny's mother sobbing so violently she was retching—a sound I'll never forget.

I remember that after Jenny died, her father insisted on helping me prepare his daughter's body for the morgue. As I began to wash Jenny, he climbed into the bed and took the washcloth from my hands. I started to remove her IVs and her father stopped me. "I want to do everything," he said, his eyes dry and dark, his voice firm. I stood back and watched as Jenny's father gently removed the tubes, the catheters. I helped as he wrapped her body in the plastic morgue bag, and I handed him the tags to tie on her toe and on the outside of the at-last-zippered-shut black shroud.

Did I kill Jenny? No, I tell myself. In my heart I know she was going to die, no matter what anyone did or didn't do. Instead I tell myself that I learned a lot that night. And one thing I learned was that sorrow comes when we least expect it, right in the middle of happiness. I learned most of all, perhaps, about grieving, about letting the survivors crawl into bed with their loved ones and *take part*, if that's what they need to do, or letting them, like Jenny's mother, get as far away as they can and *not* take part. I learned that we nurses, we caregivers, can be well trained and efficient, and yet there will always be times when we doubt our actions: Did I — the one who thought she'd done it all by graduation — give that medication too quickly, bringing Jenny's heart to a crashing halt? Did I give it too slowly, and so fail to bring her heart rate down in time?

The rest of that first night in charge is now mostly a blur. I know that the other patients lived through the night, and so did the nurse's aide and I. The post-op patient voided, coughed, and sat in a chair. The other ventilator patients were suctioned, turned, medicated, bathed, rubbed, and talked to. The patients with new MIs had no arrhythmias and received their medications on time. No IVs infiltrated or went dry. As dawn came to the unit, the sun arriving as a pale yellow line beneath the closed window shades, I sat with one man, balanced on the edge of his bed, and talked to him about his family and his business. I watched as his heart rhythm slowed and steadied, helped by 15 minutes of casual and reassuring conversation.

I can't tell you how many times in the years since that night that I've looked up the medication I gave Jenny, its properties, its side effects, its benefits, and its dangers. I can't tell you how many times since then I've stopped myself before giving a medication or a treatment to check and make sure that what the doctor ordered was correct—doctors make mistakes, too. I've learned that we caregivers are not infallible, but only as human and sometimes as frightened as our patients. We're rarely as "in charge" as we may want to believe.

That long-ago night made me a better nurse; it taught me the need for abiding caution mixed with confidence. Such caution has made me a safer nurse, especially today when everything has become more complex—how we do things, how we record things, how we interact with our patients and treat their diseases.

Still, I think about the small and mostly insignificant mistakes we make, because we are human, every day that we care for patients—all of us, from the most famous and proficient doctor to the least experienced nurse's aide. No matter the reality of what actually happens, we caregivers always carry, along with our many responsibilities, the heavy and inevitable burden of doubt.

If I've ever done anything wrong, I pray that my patients might forgive me. If there is nothing to forgive, then I wonder whether I can ever stop believing that there might be, and forgive myself.

Whistle Over the Rainbow

~

Patricia Coates Kavanaugh, RN, BSN

Dad was ever-present in my life. Mom had worked evening shifts in the 1950s. That put my father pretty high in the running to be the original "Mr. Mom."

He attended my Girl Scout functions and PTA meetings and walked to the neighborhood drugstore for medication for menstrual cramps. He encouraged me through nursing school, always ready to quiz me on what seemed to be hundreds of medication index cards. He taught me stick-shift driving on my first car, a 1970 VW Beetle, so I could drive to the university hospital no matter what shift I worked.

We had in-depth discussions about death and dying when I attended a conference with Dr. Elizabeth Kübler-Ross. We critiqued her book *On Death and Dying*. We followed her research and writings, learning and sharing our experiences. We took comfort in her belief that hearing is the last sense to leave the dying. Dad shared with me his experiences assisting with embalming at homes, a job he had in his teens. He noted that dying was a sacred time and a critical time for learning about life. He believed that when someone close to you dies, it is difficult for the living to go on living. The best way one can do that is by living without regret.

Dad cared for my children when I continued my quest for higher education. My father was there for me. In the final months of his life, I was able to be there for him. He came to live with me and my family.

I was amazed at the priceless gifts my father gave to all of us. I was reaffirmed of my husband's love, for he took care of my dad with such tenderness on weekends when I worked, always making sure he was bathed, dressed, and comfortable.

I savored each day by learning something new about my father. I found out that his first kiss was not with my mother, his wife of 53 years, but a neighbor named Julia. I asked him how he had learned that World War II was over. I learned that he was almost killed by his own men. Having been on jungle patrol in Okinawa, my father was not there for the broadcast proclaiming to the proudly serving Seabees that the war was over. Instead of a ticker-tape parade and champagne, my father was showered by bullets from the guns of his own men. Luckily they missed, and he lived to share these stories. I called his remarks pearls, jewels of life and dying that he shared so humbly in those last months. His greatest teaching was "Be kind to each other."

We had buried my mother a year and a week earlier. Now that my father was in his final days, I believed that my mother would come to help him cross over to the other side of the rainbow. I shared this with my sister, who would call every day, wanting and hoping for a report on a sighting of my mother. I kept asking him if he had seen my mother yet. Finally, after many days of this inquisition, Dad asked, "Why do you keep asking me if I have seen your mother?" I refreshed his memory about the writings and experiences of people who have had dead loved ones come to assist them in this final stage of dying.

He accepted my answer without incident. Many times in my career as an oncology nurse, my clients who were dying shared with me the unconditional peace and joy they received from loved ones who were there at the time of death "to push them over the rainbow," as my beloved pastor taught me. I was anxious, anticipating my mother being near.

Two days before his death, my father summoned me into his room and asked me, "Who was whistling?"

I listened to the deafening quiet: I didn't hear a thing.

The next day, my sister, my brother, and their families gathered at my house for what would be our last Thanksgiving dinner with my father. Dad, weakened and frail, nodded his good-byes. His eyes spoke of his love for each of us. My father passed away at 1 AM in my arms.

I was blessed not only to have had him in my life but to have had my father die in my home, where angels surround and grace is ever so present. I will be comforted all the days of my life having had that experience.

While we were honoring my dad at a luncheon following the graveyard service, his sister approached me and said, "I bet your mother is whistling for your father."

Mom had been a loud whistler, signaling us home for dinner or whistling to get everyone's attention at a party. Millie was well known for her whistle.

I had missed her.
Mother was there.
She was there to help him over the rainbow.
She whistled to my father, calling him home.

The First Patient

~

Anne Webster

It was after 5 am when Mr. Stone pushed his call button. The first morning rays streaked through his window as I found him sitting straight up in bed, one hand over his chest. Even in the half-light, I could see a peculiar gray cast to his face. When he tried to speak, only a hoarse rasp came out. Nothing we'd covered in class had addressed how to care for a patient in this kind of distress, so I ran to the desk to call for help.

Student nurses weren't allowed to disturb the private admitting physicians at home. My only hope was the intern or resident on duty, who sometimes chose to be deaf to his page — that is, if he wasn't dealing with another emergency or snoring on his bunk. And I didn't have time to look for the other student, the only other person working with me. With 52 patients between us, she could have been in any patient's room.

I returned to Mr. Stone to find him even grayer, and I could only stare helplessly. He was an old farmer in the habit of rising early. Almost recovered from an operation on his shoulder a week earlier, Mr. Stone sat with me each morning in the predawn hours at the chart desk, chatting as I fought to keep my eyes open. He'd been scheduled to go home in a day or two, but now his breath came in faint shudders. His head twisted on the pillow, and his face shone with perspiration that was icy to my touch when I stroked his arm.

A thready pulse at Mr. Stone's wrist tickled my fingertips as I thought of how I had come to be in this nightmarish situation. When I'd graduated from high school in 1958, I wanted to go to college, maybe to study medicine, but my divorced mother could barely afford secretarial school. When I won a scholarship to nursing school, I snapped at it—$175 for three years of room, board, and classes.

Contrary to my hopes, being a student nurse was far from glamorous. I soon learned that nursing students provided cheap labor, staffing the hospital around the clock. Before graduation, each girl—there were no male nurses then—rotated through every department, from dietary to obstetrics, while going to class and working six days a week.

I had somehow survived the grueling routine with only six months to graduation remaining. As senior students,

my classmates and I had become adept at dispensing medicines while slightly tipsy from early dates, dodging interns
who cornered us in the kitchen at two AM, and placating
unhappy patients. Intensive care, cardiac units, and CPR
didn't yet exist, so we were on our own when we took care
of clammy-skinned men in oxygen tents, fresh postopera-
tive patients, and anything the emergency room happened
to send us. I had learned to tell the difference between
minor bleeding at a surgical site and a serious gusher and
between heartburn and coronary pain, as well as which
unordered medicines I could get away with administering
to patients. Now veterans of every department, my classmates and I thought we knew it all, but nothing had prepared me for watching a favorite patient die.

Finally not one, but two, residents ambled into the
room. Gordon, the short one, yawned, and Bill, who
stood a foot taller, rubbed his eyes like a little boy awakened from his nap. When they came around the curtain
that was screening Mr. Stone from the other patient,
their sluggishness vanished. Gordon felt for a pulse at
Mr. Stone's throat and shook his head while Bill began to
pound on his chest. "Get a cardiac needle and some epi,"
Gordon told me. I thanked God that I remembered that
"epi" was short for epinephrine, or adrenaline.

I ran for the medicine room, praying I could find what
they needed. Miraculously a four-inch needle wrapped in
autoclave paper lay in the syringe drawer, and the epinephrine was above in the cupboard, in its assigned place.
I grabbed them and ran back down the hall. Mr. Stone's

roommate, awakened by the commotion, leaned against the wall outside the door and called my name as I sped by, but I could only nod in passing.

After Gordon fitted the needle on a syringe, he held out his hand for the vial of medicine. When I reached out to give it to him, the vial slipped from my sweaty hand and rolled under the bed. I dove after it, forgetting my starched white apron. As I groped in the dark, I heard Gordon say, "Did you see the Packers play the Colts Sunday?" Then, in the same tone, he said, "Hit him again, Bill. Hit him again." I grabbed the medicine and stood, too angry to speak. How could they talk about football when my patient was dying?

With the syringe finally filled, Gordon jabbed at the middle of Mr. Stone's chest as though he were stabbing him with an ice pick. He hit a rib with the first try, and the needle arced. Cursing under his breath, he drove it into Mr. Stone's heart with the second jab and injected the adrenaline. Mr. Stone stared, unblinking, at the ceiling as the residents took turns listening with their stethoscopes. I didn't need to be told that Mr. Stone's heart had stopped beating.

I stared at the black curls tumbling over Gordon's forehead as he leaned over the patient. My eyes followed the dark bristle on his jaw to the neck of his white jacket, where smaller black curls reached up over his tee-shirt like little fingers. Despite the tears that threatened to choke me, a familiar flutter started at the base of my belly. I let go of Mr. Stone's hand, disgusted with myself.

I heard muffled weeping, and looked up. Mr. Stone's son had stopped by on his way to work, and there he stood, staring at his father's still body. A wave of guilt washed over me. Mr. Stone's well-being had been in my hands, yet he had died. I knew I should say something to his son, put my arm around his shoulders, and get him some tissues, but my own eyes were filling with tears. I fled the room, dodging the other patient as I ran past, and hid, trembling, behind the medicine room door.

None of our teachers had ever told us about losing a patient, about how quickly someone could go from being a jolly person to a dead body. Nor had they warned of the nagging sense of inadequacy and failure that would haunt me for weeks afterward. During my 25-year nursing career, I became almost blasé about death, yet even now, I feel a twinge of guilt, wondering if I could have done something more to save Mr. Stone.

Combing Her Hair

~

Mary DeLisle-Berry, RN

I KNOCKED ON THE DOOR and a man answered. He invited me in. His name, he said, was Hank. He was the husband of the patient I was going to meet for the first time that day.

I am a registered nurse, and I had been assigned as the case manager for a 56-year-old woman named Maryanne. She had a diagnosis of pancreatic cancer. Hank told me his wife was upstairs and asked if I would like a cup of coffee before I went up to meet her.

I like to get to know the family early into my relationship with my clients. Hospice is a collaborative venture with the patient, family, and hospice staff. Hospice provides the teaching and the medical supplies needed for end-of-life care. Nursing, social work, chaplaincy, and volunteer staff offer physical, emotional, and spiritual care and support when they visit. But family and friends are the primary care providers. They are the ones there 24/7 to meet the daily needs of the patient and support that person through the dying process. They likely will be at the bedside when their loved one dies; they will dial the phone and make the call to hospice when that happens.

I sat down and took my coffee with cream, and Hank and I chatted. He was a nice man. Quite a talker. I don't really recall what we talked about. After about ten minutes or so of small talk, I thanked him for the coffee, got up from the kitchen table, and went up the stairs to meet his wife. I had no idea then what an adventure I had ahead of me. It forever changed my life, deepening my awareness of the power of love.

Maryanne was a matter-of-fact, "don't-bullshit-me" woman. She asked me, "How long do I have to live?" shortly after my Avon-lady "Hi, my name is Mary. I'm your hospice nurse" intro. Okay, I thought, apparently no time was going to be spent here in chitchatting with Maryanne.

When I mentioned how I enjoyed meeting her husband Hank, she said that I had talked more with Hank in the last ten minutes than she had in the last ten years. Interesting, I thought, particularly because Hank ultimately was going to assume the role of primary caregiver.

I stumbled through that first visit with Maryanne—she was very guarded. No touchy-feely stuff wafting in the air. No hand-holding. She wanted a schedule of when

I would be visiting, a list of the meds she would be taking, and to be kept informed about how long she had to live and how she would die; she specifically wanted to know what would happen physiologically that would cause her death. "Don't spare any details," she instructed. So we made a schedule for my visits, we reviewed her medications, and I agreed to be totally honest and straightforward with the information she wanted from me. She had clearly defined what she wanted from hospice; I was clearly committed to providing hospice care for her—her way. The dance had begun.

Early in my visits with Maryanne, during every visit she was very insistent that I increase the dose of her morphine and Ativan. I would bring her request to our hospice doctor, and her pain and anti-anxiety medications were increased. Pain and anxiety are what the patient says they are, and hospice is about meeting comfort needs and managing pain. But during my visits after these increases in dosage, all I ever observed was my patient getting more and more "dopey."

On one of these visits she slurred out the question, "How long 'til I die?" I'd gotten to know her well enough by then that I felt I knew how to answer that one. We had actually established a good rapport and had discussed many of her beliefs about life and death. So I said, "Well, unless you drown from drooling, or pass out and fall into your oatmeal and meet the same fate, I suspect it is going to be awhile yet." That woke her up a bit.

I explained graphically, as I agreed at the beginning I

would, that physiologically her body still had fat to burn and it had the ability to use that fat for energy. Her body was not burning muscle yet. Her heart was a muscle, and it was strong. I was speaking her language. I knew we were connecting. "You are not leaving anytime soon as far as I can see," I said. She got teary-eyed.

It wasn't physical pain she was trying to get rid of; it was fear she was trying to medicate away. She said so after my seemingly rude and to-the-point reply to her question. It was an effective pattern interrupt. And she got it. What she was doing was not working. I then asked her if she would like to explore a few other ways to manage some of this fear. She said yes. And I believe at that point hospice spun its magic, and the dignity and grace Maryanne and Maryanne's family deserved to experience at her end-of-life journey began.

Maryanne belonged to the Baha'i faith. Friends from her congregation would come to visit. They brought food and little gifts of inspirational readings to offer support to her. She had been involved for years with the Baha'i faith and was a very active member in their local community. She told me she had always found strength and purpose through integrating her faith into her everyday life. But when she was diagnosed with cancer, her entire focus had gotten stuck on the question of when and how she would die.

She wasn't able to take in the love and comfort from her friends. When they came over she was "drugged." She was unable to quiet her mind long enough to think about anything else. Her actually physical pain was managed very well. Her spiritual pain was raging, but her source for addressing that pain was blocked. None of the drugs she was taking could manage that kind of pain.

Because she had agreed to try some alternative symptom management, I suggested guided imagery. Perhaps she could relax, and that might open a pathway for her to quiet her mind and find strength again in the things that had sustained her throughout her life. She was very receptive to that idea. She had used hypnosis many years prior to quit smoking and was pleased at how well that had worked for her.

A session of guided imagery was held at her bedside and taped for her; it was scripted by her, for her, specifically using her favorite imaginings: Thoughts and ideas that brought her peace of mind and hope were used to help her remember how she had lived her life before fear had taken over.

I remember very well one story she wanted on that tape to help her relax: Maryanne said her father was a fisherman. When she was a little girl she would sit on the dock and watch for him to come in with his boat at the end of the day. It was a carefree time in her life, when she felt safe and loved. So that is the story we used to promote relaxation on the tape. We put some of her favorite poems and songs and spiritual quotes into the tape as well. It was her tape, done her way. She loved it! She listened to it when she felt anxious, when she went to sleep at night, when she wanted to catnap during the day. She fell into the experience of relaxing with it. And slowly over the weeks that followed, she had us wean her medications down to levels that managed her pain and yet allowed her to be present and alert for her life. She started enjoying the visits from her friends. She was even talking to Hank. One day when I came to visit, Hank was combing her hair. It made me cry.

Not all of my experiences in hospice have been so dramatic, but they have all been unique and sacred. Seeing "don't-bullshit-me" Maryanne having her hair brushed by a man she said she had barely spoken to in the past ten years touched me deeply. Later, after her death, when I met her two grown daughters, they told me of some very amazing conversations they had with their mom during those months prior to her death. They told me how stunned they were observing the tenderness between their parents during that time. One daughter said her mom and dad seemed to have fallen in love again—something she never thought she would see.

I honestly do not know how all that healing happened between them. I'm guessing Maryanne and Hank must have called a truce at one point to the silence and done some talking with each other. He had become her caregiver, bathing her, helping to feed her, and sitting vigil many hours at her bedside. It was Hank who made the call to hospice when she died.

What I do know is that Maryanne knew what she needed to do to make peace with her life and her death. She was stuck, and hospice brought some ideas in to help her get through the stuckness so she could tap her own

It's Heaven I See

~

Angela Posey-Arnold, RN, BSN

ONCE A YEAR, just one time a year, I left the facility where I served as director of nursing. Once a year, I hoped that it would run on autopilot. My administrator and I would leave the facility for one week in May to attend the Alabama State Nursing Home Convention in Gulf Shores, Alabama. It was a learning vacation, but I always felt a little guilty about leaving my staff and residents.

One year, I meticulously checked and rechecked all my 103 residents several times before I left. I made sure the staff had what they needed, and I left the assistant director of nursing and the physician assistant in charge. I prepared to be gone for two weeks before I left. I had confidence in my nursing administration team, my licensed practical nurses, and my certified nursing assistants. I knew they could handle anything that could arise. The

LPNs were all in place and the CNAs were the best there were. I felt secure the facility would run smoothly.

Two days into the conference, having gotten just a little bit of a tan, I received an urgent message in the middle of a meeting. I went out of the meeting and called my assistant director of nursing. She was in tears.

"Angela, you have to come home. Titus died. He just died. What are we going to do?"

It wasn't that she didn't know what the procedure was following the death of a resident. It was that she knew the entire staff, from nursing to housekeeping, would be devastated by his sudden and seemingly untimely death.

Titus was a gentle, loving soul in his late fifties. He had been a brittle diabetic for years and was on dialysis. Most days he felt pretty good and on days he didn't feel good, he faked it. He always tried to be positive and encouraging to other people. He was more of a helper in the facility than a resident. He spent his time talking to other residents, especially the new ones. He would help the new ones get adjusted and was the first friend they made in their new surroundings. He loved the nurses and we loved him. When things happened at the facility, he would be among the first ones at my door offering to help. I usually put him to work helping in some way that he could.

He didn't have any family that visited. Titus had one brother, but he had never come to see him. It didn't bother Titus—he was surrounded by family. He was with his family every day. We were his family.

His death was sudden and unexpected. The night-shift nurse went in to wake him and found him dead. He had died peacefully in his sleep. My assistant director of nursing reported that Titus had the most peaceful smile on his face. He had a strong faith in God and talked about how wonderful heaven would be. No more finger sticks, no more dialysis, no more amputations: He looked forward to it. He always told me that Jesus was his best friend.

The assistant director of nursing had called the doctor and the physician's assistant was on his way. The nurse had done everything required as far as procedure goes, but when the day shift arrived, everyone was so upset. We were all upset. We had lost a member of our family, and I was away.

Those that are not blessed to work in long-term care might think that we deal with death on a daily basis. We don't. Long-term care is just that—long term. It is not a place to go to die; it is a place to go to live. If a resident becomes acutely and seriously ill, the doctor usually sends that person to the hospital.

At this very difficult time, my administrator and I were 600 miles from home. One of our beloved had died suddenly and unexpectedly. He had been doing very well before I left. He had assured me that he would take care of everything, and then smiled that sweet smile. We considered going back home, but we had already signed up and paid for the conference. We really couldn't leave.

So over the phone, I counseled several CNAs and LPNs, who were just crushed. As sad as we all were by Titus's death, I was so proud of my nurses. I was proud of them because they cared so deeply. They were not afraid to love our residents and through that love, they provided excellent care.

In February of that year, we had all collected money and bought Titus a brand-new suit: blue pinstripe, with a white shirt and a red tie that he picked out. He looked so handsome in his new suit. The smile on his face was radiant. He had been elected King for Valentine's Day, and we always made a big deal out of that.

To Titus it was a big deal. I remember the day he found out that he had won.

He said with tears in his eyes, "I've never had such an honor."

He looked so handsome in his new suit, but he refused to wear it any other time. He said he was saving it for a big date.

The staff had his suit cleaned and pressed, and one of them took it to the funeral home for him to be buried in. The Activities director took a picture from the Valentine's Day celebration and had it enlarged and framed for the guest book table.

None of us knew Titut's brother, but he took care of the burial expenses. He asked us to make the arrangements.

The CNA who had cared for Titus for 15 years made the arrangements. Visitation was from 2 o'clock until 4 o'clock so all shifts could attend. The funeral was set for Sunday at two PM. Staff was pulled in from the part-time pool so that most everyone that wanted to go could attend. Some of the residents attended, too, brought by their families. The funeral was held by our chaplain, and the nurses were seated in the family section. Titus's favorite hymns were played, and as they closed the casket one of the CNAs sang "I Can See Clearly Now."

It was all over by the time my administrator and I returned to the facility. The front lobby and the nurse's desk were overflowing with flowers from the funeral. We later had a memorial service at the facility, during which everyone who wanted to say a few words about Titus could do so. We planted a new flower bed in his memory. He had always loved planting flowers and watching them grow. When they were in full bloom, he would pick a fresh bouquet for each nurse's desk. The memorial service was something we all needed for closure together. We laughed, we cried, and we healed.

We had a plaque made and placed on the hall where Titus had lived for 15 years. Inscribed in the plaque was his name, date of birth, date of death, and the words "Don't Cry for Me. It's Heaven I See."

Healing had begun. I was somewhat concerned that the nurses would be afraid to love again, but they weren't. The experience strengthened their bond together. It strengthened the bond we had with them. They kept right on loving and providing exceptional nursing care every single day. The trial had strengthened their character. They became even better nurses. When a new nurse was hired, she quickly found out about our Titus and how special he was to us all.

He is still remembered with a smile as the nurses continue to love; even though they know they may get their hearts broken, the love never fails. Compassionate nursing and long-term care go hand in hand.

It doesn't matter whether you can start insert a PICC line in five seconds flat—if you don't have compassion and the ability to put your heart out there and love your patients, you have missed a very wonderful part of nursing. Compassion is the most important quality a nurse can have.

Fatal Catheter

≈

Patrick D. Colwell, RN

Most patients let you know one way or another that the insertion of the catheter is not their favorite part of the day. A catheter is a sterile rubber tube used for emptying the urinary bladder when the patient is unable to manage that task himself. It also may be used to obtain a sterile urine sample for laboratory analysis. A catheter can be "straight," meaning it is inserted once, then removed and discarded, or "Foley," which has an inflatable balloon on the end to hold it in the bladder for a period of time. The only people grateful to have a catheter inserted are the ones who come to the emergency room with a bladder ready to burst. Inability to empty the bladder sometimes happens after a surgery. My guess is the general anesthetic sedates some parts of the body before others.

Dr. Miller first came to our emergency room as a resident, which is when I met her. On that occasion, she asked me to please call her by her first name. This may sound odd, but I told her I didn't think I could do that. I will write more about the special relationship that exists between doctors and nurses who work well together, but for now I will mention just two things. First, I always addressed Dr. Miller and all of the ER docs as "Doctor" because I wanted to communicate my very real respect for them, especially when patients were present. I was afraid that addressing them by their first names would become a habit that would manifest itself accidentally. Consequently I can recall Dr. Miller's face, her sense of humor, and many of the things she said, but I honestly cannot recall her first name.

The second reason I used the title "Doctor" was to avoid, under other circumstances, getting my face ripped off and handed to me. That would not occur with our ER docs, but on that great totem pole of rank in health care, a nurse should avoid presumption.

Despite my use of formal title, Dr. Miller and I got off to a playful start. She frequently displayed a great sense of humor. I recall that I had to ask her a couple of times to sign her written orders, and it got to be a joke between us. I enjoyed trying to catch those few occasions when she absentmindedly left the signature line of the physician's order blank, and she enjoyed depriving me of the satisfaction of catching her. Dr. Miller was in her early thirties when I knew her, quite a number of years younger than I was. She was married and had a teenage daughter. From time to time she made some interesting remarks.

In our ER, the nurses usually assess the patient before the physician sees the chart or the patient. One afternoon I was briefly describing a rather taciturn, nearly immobile female patient with vague complaints I no longer recall.

"I'm not sure exactly why she's here," I told Dr. Miller. "She doesn't give me much. She just sort of lays there."

The doctor smiled and looked me right in the eye. Loud enough for several coworkers to overhear, she said, "So you're saying it was like having sex."

I spent three seconds in stunned silence, wondering whether I had really heard that or had hallucinated. Keeping my facial expression as serious as I could manage, I replied, "No, actually, I'm not saying that."

Another time I walked by Dr. Miller's desk just as she said to someone else, "That's why God gave the breasts to women." Then she turned that mischievous smile on me. "If you guys had those you'd never leave home."

How did she know? I thought that was a secret.

Statistically our ER has a cyclical patient load that exactly matches the U.S. average for emergency departments. That means we have too many patients nearly every day, but Sundays are the worst. If you have been a parent, you know that kids always seem to get sick on the weekend, when their doctor's office is closed. Also, many people are off work on the weekend, engaging in recreational activities. I have a low opinion of motorized recreation, based on some unpleasant realities I encountered in the ER. If a person is at work, then he does not have the chance to fall off his four-wheeler and fracture, say, his humerus. If he is at work, he does not roll his four-wheeler and trigger a cerebral hemorrhage that fries his brain. He also does not fall off the back of the four-wheeler and land on the daughter who was seated behind him. Nor does he, while at work, drive his four-wheeler 38 miles per hour *in reverse* and roll it, fracturing his femur. Nope: He does all those things on the weekend.

I don't know for certain, but my gut feeling is that more people get shot and stabbed on weekends, especially since they get drunk, stoned, and high more often on Friday and Saturday than on weekdays. Of course, physicians' offices are closed on Sundays, and the police do not haul their handcuffed out-of-control methamphetamine and cocaine abusers to the local urgent care center. All of these factors combined can make the 12-hour weekend shifts in a busy ER a real trial for those who work there.

One particular Sunday stands out in my mind as the busiest I have ever experienced. We had patients in every available bed, not only in rooms but in the hallways, by the nurses' locker room, by the ambulance garage, and across from the cast room. We had patients sitting upright in chairs because we ran out of beds. There were patients waiting in the lobby, becoming more and more short-tempered about the wait. I'm told that in large U.S. cities, patients frequently wait six hours to see an ER physician. Although our wait time did not tend to be that lengthy, I will mention that on Sundays like the one I am describing, an independent observer might just say that something was a bit off kilter in the American health care system.

The ambulances never stopped rolling in that day. Ideally, we liked to "clean up the board" for the next shift, meaning we admit to an inpatient room or discharge to home as many patients as possible to give the next shift as decent a start as possible. On this shift, we labored hard all day and still handed the next shift a chaotic mess.

One of the ambulances brought us a patient from the hospice organization for the terminally ill. This 80-something gentleman suffered from dementia, advanced cardiac disease, kidney problems, and other ailments. His wife, daughter, and hospice nurse arrived about the same time as the ambulance. I learned all of his history from the family and the nurse, because this poor man could not accurately answer questions anymore. The problem that brought him to us that day was inability to empty his urinary bladder. The hospice nurse had tried to insert a catheter, but she was unable to get it in. As he lay on our bed he was quite uncomfortable. He could verify that he hurt, but his speech didn't make much sense otherwise.

Concerned about the patient's advanced heart disease, I spoke to his daughter and wife: "I want to make sure I understand something. If his heart or his breathing stops while he is here, do you want us to try to bring him back?"

The daughter looked me in the eye and said, "Absolutely not." His wife shifted her gaze uncomfortably away from me, but agreed with her daughter. I wrote the abbreviation "DNR," for "do not resuscitate," in large letters on the first page of his chart.

I hustled through the crammed hallway to the nurses' station and spoke to Dr. Miller about this patient. I reasoned that we might be able to quickly "treat and street" this one if she would order me to place a catheter before seeing the patient herself. As I recall she elected to see the patient first, but also told me to go ahead and get the equipment because she would be in the patient's room for only a few minutes.

I grabbed a Foley kit and a coudee catheter from the supply closet. Then I found Bradley and recruited him to help me. Bradley is an emergency medical technician intermediate level. This means Bradley can start IVs in our ER under nurse supervision. The supervision works like this: The nurse yells across the room, "Bradley! Can you go start an IV on Room 4?" Bradley, Jerry, and Ted (the latter two are paramedics, a step above EMT intermediate) are like gold. They are super workers, they're completely trustworthy, and they have great senses of humor. On this occasion I needed Bradley to help me get the catheter in because the patient would be unable to cooperate in his state of confusion.

Bradley and I entered Room 14 as Dr. Miller left. I asked the family whether they wanted to stay or step outside while we attempted to insert the catheter. They opted to step out, as did the hospice nurse. We shut the door and pulled the privacy curtain in case someone opened the door. I briefly explained to our patient what we were going to do. I don't think he understood, but I recall he was polite to us. I've observed that the dying process may reveal a person's real personality, depending on what that person's illness is. Strip away my ability to think clearly, and whatever I am really like is what you will see. In this case a very confused, kind gentleman was still kind when he could not understand what was happening to him. Some diseases may alter the dying person's personality, I am sure. Other times you simply see what is really there.

We uncovered him below the waist. I opened the kit and donned the sterile gloves while Bradley pulled on clean exam gloves and steadied the patient's legs. Bradley was ready to hold firmly if the patient decided to kick or fight. I cleaned the patient per protocol. Because the hospice nurse had been unable to get a catheter in, I decided to use a trick I learned from experienced nurses during my student days: I injected the syringe of sterile lubricant from the kit directly into the patient's urethra. With older men the prostate gland is frequently enlarged, making it difficult to pass a catheter all the way from the urethral opening into the bladder. The prostate squeezes the urethra, and in fact may be the cause of the urinary retention. Standard catheter insertion calls for lubricating just the tip of the catheter before inserting it. Experience has taught me that injecting the lubricant sometimes works better. If I couldn't insert the catheter that way, my plan was to try the coudee, which is a catheter with a semi-rigid tip. If the coudee also failed, I could ask another nurse to try. If that failed as well, we would let Dr. Miller know. In some cases of this nature, I've known ER docs to call a urologist, reasoning that if two ER nurses could not get the catheter in, then it was time to call a specialist. On this day, Plan A worked. After a few minutes of manipulating the catheter into our patient's well-lubricated urethra, I got it past the prostate and into the bladder. The telltale sign of success is a flow of urine through the tubing and into the bag attached to the sterile catheter. I have to admit I felt a small rush of satisfaction. Undoubtedly, the hospice nurse was very experienced at this, but I had Bradley helping me while she had probably worked alone.

As mentioned, this gentleman was nice to us even in his advanced state of illness and confusion. Despite that, when I inserted the catheter, it hurt him. He cried out and tried to sit up, clenching his eyes shut. Bradley and I tried to soothe him, telling him it would hurt for only a few minutes. We told him it would be less painful if he could lie back and relax. He did lie back on the bed. Next he started talking, and this time it made sense.

"All right, that's it!" he said forcefully, his eyes still shut tightly. "I'm all through, Jesus, that's it."

I looked at Bradley, who looked back at me.

"Jesus, forgive me for everything. Just forgive me for everything, all my sins," he went on. I won't pretend to recall what he said word for word, but he repeated it several times. The gist was "That's it, I've had enough. Jesus, forgive me for all my sins."

"Do you think he's really talking to Jesus?" I asked Bradley.

"I think he is."

We finished our procedure, covered him back up, and tried to make him as comfortable as we could. By the time his wife and daughter and the hospice nurse returned, his speech was once again quite confused. The hospice nurse was very nice to me. "You actually got a catheter in him! I'm impressed." I reported the success to Dr. Miller, thinking she would discharge him immediately. Then I got caught up in some other case.

Quite frankly, I forgot all about my urinary retention patient until about 45 minutes later. We had several critically ill patients in the department. Earlier that day, the fire and rescue guys brought us a code blue patient who had died. With one thing and another going on, Dr. Miller had gotten tied up. She had not yet discharged our patient with the recently emptied bladder and the indwelling Foley catheter. As I hustled past Room 14, the hospice nurse grabbed my arm.

"Something is wrong," she said curtly. "He's not breathing right."

I entered the room with her reluctantly. The old fellow had turned gray in the face. His breathing was irregular, almost gasping.

I looked at the hospice nurse. "I think he's going now."

"I think so, too."

I walked quickly to the noisy, crammed, bustling nurses' station knowing I could not politely wait my turn.

"Dr. Miller," I said fairly loudly over the top of all the other noise, "Room 14 is dying right now. He's a DNR."

She hesitated for half a second, then walked ahead of me to Room 14. We closed the door and stood there with the patient's wife and daughter. In that room, we had a few quiet moments as we watched him leave this world. His pulse got weaker and slower, and his breathing slowed to once every 20 or 30 seconds. A couple of times, when I thought he was gone, he startled me by taking another agonizing breath. I had the urge to thrust his jaw upward to open the airway, but I did not. I just felt his pulse and looked at my watch to time the last few breaths of his life. Someone, somewhere, eight decades earlier had watched him take his first breath as a newborn babe. I watched him take his very last breath in this world.

"That's it," he had said less than an hour before he died, "I'm all done. Jesus, forgive me for everything."

Dr. Miller was very kind to the family. His wife, in her eighties like her husband, sat on one of our chairs crying. "I knew this was coming but it's still hard," she sobbed. Dr. Miller put her arm around the poor woman and told her how sorry she was. She also said he was not suffering anymore.

About 30 minutes later, another of Dr. Miller's critically ill patients died, bringing the department total to three that day. As we stood in the unrelenting din of the nurses' station I saw her throw her hands in the air and say, "God, what's it like to actually cure somebody?"

We were not having our best day ever. I had been

primary nurse on the earlier code blue, so I was tied up for quite a while processing the stack of paperwork that attends an unsuccessful resuscitation. Then my urinary retention DNR patient had died. I asked Paula, who had been an ER nurse far longer than I, whether three deaths was a record for a shift.

"I don't think so," she said. "There was the time the bar exploded." I didn't want to know, on second thought.

Meanwhile, we were still getting hammered by too many patients and not enough rooms. After Room 14's family left, we covered his body and moved it to the hazmat room, which typically was used to store equipment related to hazardous material spills. It sounds callous, but we desperately needed Room 14. The mortician had not yet come for the body.

About this time I overheard Karla, our nurse in charge, holding half of a tense phone conversation with a nurse on an inpatient floor. She hung up the phone. Apparently in the melee of the late afternoon Tracy, our unit clerk, had sent that unit one of our patients when a bed was ready. Normally a nurse would make the transfer. Tracy was trying to help out, knowing that we were all buried up to the eyebrows in bodies, three of them dead but the rest still alive. The floor nurses were furious because no one had called report before we sent the patient to them.

Karla said, "They actually asked me, 'What if that patient had been really sick?' Imagine that! Having really sick patients to deal with! I told them I'm sorry, but we've had three deaths down here today, we've got dead bodies in our storage rooms, and we're just a little busy. We'll try to do better next time."

"Karla, I've got a great idea," I said, quickly progressing from humor to degenerating hysteria. "Let's send them a dead body. When they call up to complain that they didn't get the report we can tell them not to hurry with their assessment, since the patient is *already dead.*" We laughed our way through this bout of group mental illness.

An hour later, about hour 11 of this memorable shift, the mortician arrived to transport the body of my patient to the funeral home. As I helped him, I briefly wondered what would have happened if I'd forgotten about the body in the hazmat room and the next shift of nurses found it.

By hour 12, I was completely punchy, but deeply grateful that the nightmare shift was finally ending. I walked into the nurses' station to find Dr. Miller smiling mischievously at me, flanked by Karla and Paula. Obviously it was an ambush.

"Pat," she said, "I've come to a decision."

"What are you talking about?" I asked, wearily.

"When my time comes, I want you to cath me."

I leaned forward. "What did you say?"

I must have had a strange expression on my face. Karla and Paula burst into laughter.

"No, really," Dr. Miller insisted. "The way that guy died after you cathed him—he just sort of slid peacefully off. You have the touch. That's the way I want to go. So when it's my time, I want you to cath me."

"Lovely. I guess I'll take that as a vote of confidence," I said, as they laughed themselves hypoxic.

Carol

~

Geraldine Gorman, RN, PhD

I ONCE ARRANGED A meeting between Ted, the lanky fine arts jeweler, and Carol. Although well intentioned, it was probably a mistake. What they had in common—inquisitive minds, youthful middle age, and aggressive lung cancer—also functioned as a repellant. I can only imagine what each saw in the other on the afternoon I brought them together on the oncology unit. To my knowledge, it was their only conversation.

My own introduction to Carol was a while in coming. Long before I met her, I knew of her through bits and scraps exchanged at the nurses' station: 41 years old, diagnosed just one month after completing her doctorate in medical humanities, recent admission precipitated by a pneumothorax. The collapsed lung could be treated, but the overall prognosis was bleak. The door to her room remained closed; only Sister Grace, the Dominican nun who served as our formidable charge nurse, moved in and out. Carol was our contemporary, much younger than most who passed through our unit, and we were all a bit subdued by what must have been unfolding within her darkened room.

When she did emerge, it was with a flourish. During the Sunday evening shift, the door banged open. Out came Carol in her wheelchair, red cowboy bandana around her head, hazel eyes wide, very much alive. In her hand she held a sparkly baton, which she waved as a chorus line of women in their thirties and forties trailed behind her. Round and round they circled the nurses' station, whooping as we gawked. The occasion was Carol's five-year anniversary with Rhonda, pointed out to me by Elizabeth, my recent preceptor, as the stocky woman with the gravelly laugh who piloted the wheelchair. Work on the oncology unit came to a momentary halt in deference to such a rare spectacle.

As Carol emerged more fully into our world, nurses other than Grace took over her care. Throughout the early weeks of October, as she recuperated and regained strength, we came to know one another. Revelations spawned affection. For a brief intersection of time, Carol and I forged a friendship, deeply, heedlessly.

That I had been an English major delighted her. We swapped favorites: Flannery O'Connor short stories, Eugene O'Neill plays. Neither of us could say too much about contemporary poetry, so we backed up: Yeats and Eliot and Stevens and, of course, Plath and Sexton. Feminist polemics were a given: Greer and Millet and Chernin. In 1992, I had been out of graduate school for 13 years; "postmodern" was not a whisper in our academic jargon when I graduated. Carol obligingly offered me some new and exotic names for my reading list: Foucault and Derrida, Iragary and Cixoux. Her dissertation argued that physicians could increase their empathetic response and success rate with alcoholic patients by becoming better versed in the humanities, and she had explicit suggestions for them. For her structural framework she employed a hologram, a fact I found interesting but could not fully appreciate until embroiled in my own dissertation woes years later. She taught med students at a couple of Midwestern universities and she had big plans. When I brought her a picture my daughter Grace drew for her, Carol promptly named Grace illustrator of her next book. "We will all collaborate; it'll be great," she promised. "Egghead!" growled Rhonda from her chair in the corner. "You are all eggheads."

Dr. Patel served as Carol's oncologist and when she asked me what I thought of him, I hedged. I'd been on the unit only a few months and, from what I had observed thus far, was unimpressed. I certainly had no other options to offer, however, so I remained noncommittal. Carol was not particularly interested in bedside manner; she slept as much as she could manage between treatments and just wanted the most expedient route to getting the hell out. Her chemotherapy protocol was the one typically utilized for lung carcinoma. Beyond that, there remained little I could tell her. Besides, she was my friend. The nursing role began to chafe a bit, though I was not sure why. I knew only that I never wanted to hang her chemo, and as fate and schedules converged, I was never called upon to do so.

Once Carol recovered from the pneumothorax and was discharged, she began her stint as an outpatient. She came to the clinic dressed always in gray sweats and, having discarded the bandanas, her hazel eyes compelled all the more, dominating such a streamlined countenance. One of her many devoted friends accompanied her; usually it was Kate, an aspiring politician with a gentle voice and a sad, knowing look. Carol remained unabashedly squeamish about needles, jumpy and decidedly non-stoic regarding anything she perceived as an assault upon her body. The sparkly baton I first observed at her coming-out party I soon came to know as her "cancer stick," and she waved it wildly in the face of anyone preparing to foist upon her person what she considered to be an odious act.

After months of sustained chemo, her veins gave out. With it becoming more and more difficult to gain venous access, Sister Grace and her legion of friends began the Herculean task of convincing her to permit a central line that would allow her battered blood vessels respite. The installation of the "port-a-cath"—a small repository located near her heart through which the drugs could be administered—required an overnight stay. Her pre-op care fell to me. She arrived in a state of high anxiety that only escalated. She told jokes and laughed; she held

Rhonda's hand and cried. Squirming and fidgeting and glaring at her friends who sat calmly devouring cinnamon buns from the famous Scandinavian restaurant in their neighborhood, she finally exhausted their patience. Kate found me in the corridor. "Isn't there something you can give her to take the edge off?" she asked. There was, but it came in a syringe.

I entered Carol's room, steeling myself for the bartering session. She finally acquiesced to the Demerol. As I retrieved the medication, I paused: Shit. This was not going to be easy. And it wasn't. Carol demanded to see the syringe and blanched. Then she withdrew permission. She would not allow it. I waited. Okay, okay, I could do it; I just had to give her a minute. She scrunched up her face and whimpered. She started to pull down the blanket but changed her mind.

"Oh, God," she said, "Oh God."

"Jesus Christ, honey, it's just a damn shot. Go ahead, give it to her," announced Rhonda, steadying Carol's arm.

I uncapped the syringe and stabbed the needle into her deltoid. She howled. Once the surgery was successfully completed and the port-a-cath in place, she was content and playful as a kitten. What a great idea, she conceded.

Following my departure from the hospital I stayed in contact with Carol, though I saw her less frequently. In mid-March she invited me to a board game party she and Rhonda were hosting at their condominium. Parking proved scarce in their increasingly trendy northside neighborhood and I walked blocks through a warm but steady drizzle. Card tables in the living room, dining room, and den offered a choice of Parcheesi, Monopoly, Clue, checkers, chess, backgammon, and assorted card games. Laughing women moved from tables to kitchen, filling their plates with chili from the crockpot, chips and guacamole, goat cheese and crackers, and chocolate cookies of various shapes and sizes, with nuts and without. A few men from the neighborhood drifted in and out, sipping red wine and kibitzing with the ladies. Carol was in the middle of everything, sometimes standing, mostly sitting. She gave me a tour, ending with her study. "This," she pointed in triumph, "is where I finished the damn dissertation." I imagined her sitting there, smoking and writing, as Rhonda supplied the coffee and kept the outside world at bay.

Carol was buoyant and boisterous but notably thinner. They were growing increasingly impatient with Dr. Patel, with his well-honed evasiveness, and the toxicity of the side effects of treatment. Encouraged by members of the Lesbian Health Alliance, Carol added Chinese herbs and acupuncture to her medicinal arsenal.

When I announced my departure, she grabbed my hand and walked me down the long hall to the door. The gesture caught me off guard—it was such a sweetly un–self-conscious pajama-party thing to do—and the thought washed over me: *Oh God, my friend, my friend Carol. Let her be okay, please, just let her be okay.* At the door she thanked me for coming and for giving her the piece

I had written following my father's recent death. "I've got this friend, a physician in the Medical Humanities department at Iowa. You should send it to him," she said, and she wrote the name down on a slip of paper. I asked about the dry cough that came and went, convulsing her slender frame. "It's nothing," she said. "Just a cold I can't shake." We embraced, and I headed home to fix dinner for my waiting children.

I was standing at the sink, washing dishes and watching the setting sun play off the roof of the public school outside my kitchen window. It was mid-June and unseasonably cool. The phone rang and my daughter Grace called me. On the line, Rhonda's husky voice shook: They could not rouse Carol and she didn't know what to do. She had promised her no more hospitals, but she just wasn't sure now. Could I come?

Rhonda briefed me when I arrived. Carol had been rapidly declining. That day they had gone to see a homeopathic practitioner, one of the few routes they had not yet tried. He took one look at her and sent them home. Carol went to bed, and now they could not wake her. In the darkened living room, Kate sat by herself, Kleenex wadded in her hand. Rhonda accompanied me to the bedroom. Carol lay on her back, mouth slack, breathing deeply. She was obtunded—flesh drawn so tightly over swollen tissue that I barely recognized her. But when I sat on the bed and withdrew the blood pressure cuff from my bag, her eyes flew open. "Hi, honey," she said. Unmistakably Carol.

Her blood pressure was tanking: 90/60. Her heart raced: 110 beats per minute. She was hot to the touch, with a temperature of 102. She slurred her words. Rhonda half-carried her to the bathroom, where she shook with violent diarrhea. "Oh sorry, I'm sorry," she said over and over as Rhonda murmured and stroked her cheek. Once back in bed, she returned to a deep slumber, and Rhonda and I moved to the kitchen.

From the beginning of Carol's illness, Rhonda was resolute and unflagging in her optimism and support. They would get through this. No matter what—no matter the diagnosis, the statistics, the side effects, the inscrutability of the oncologist—they would make it. Carol drew her hope from Rhonda. Standing there in the kitchen, eyes rid-rimmed, swollen, and darkened, she teetered beyond exhaustion. I told her I thought she had kept her promise of no hospitalizations when it most mattered and that now it was necessary, for her and for Carol. She raised no objection. We called the internist, a thoughtful man who had cared for Carol over the years, and admission was arranged. I went in to tell her. At first she looked at me with incomprehension. Then she said, "But I can't just give up, can I?" Rhonda returned to the bedroom. I left to sit with Kate in silent darkness till the ambulance arrived. Placing the stretcher next to the bed and pulling on their latex gloves, the emergency medical technicians asked Rhonda Carol's age. "Just 42," she answered.

CALLIE WAS ONE OF MY regular patients when I began home health care with the Visiting Nurse Association. Her cat, Pretty Kitty, was a hulking mass of a feline. Each time I visited Callie to administer her calcitonin injection for her severe osteoporosis, I battled with the cat, half petting her, half shoving her away from my nursing bag. I was thus engaged in Callie's kitchen when my pager went off. I called the oncology unit and Terry, the licensed practical nurse, told me Carol had just died.

I had been to visit her two days before, 48 hours after her late-night admission. It was my first return to the hospital since leaving in January, and I wanted to see as few people as possible. Carol's room was near the staircase, so I walked up the five flights and ducked in quickly. Her friends had transformed the private room into their own facsimile of a feminist hospice. Candles burned on the windowsill, sandalwood incense scented the room. Carol's friends rubbed her swollen limbs with lavender oil. At the head of the bed sat Rhonda, her complexion sallow, eyes swollen, voice reduced to a whisper. Sister Grace was the only nurse to venture in, just as had been the case when Carol first came to the unit, almost exactly a year before. The Dominican nun tended her with gentle affection, but she remained ever the school principal, instructing the assembled ladies on protocol for the dying. "Keep talking to her," she told them. "Hearing is the last sense to diminish. But let her know it is okay for her to go." And offering a demonstration, Sister Grace leaned over Carol. "It is all right to go now, dear. We love you, but God is waiting for you." Carol's eyes flew open. "Can we talk about this?" she said.

I stood at the foot of the bed watching Rhonda caress her head. There had not been sufficient time between, or after, chemotherapy sessions for her hair to return, so she remained as I had always known her—sparse, no adornments, the essence of Carol burning through her eyes. She would murmur occasionally and then return to soporific depths. When Rhonda whispered in her ear, "Look, honey, look who has come to see you. It's Gerry," her eyes fluttered and she responded, "Hi, honey, hi, honey." After several minutes of silence, Carol became momentarily agitated. She turned her head toward Rhonda and tried to sit up. "Kitties, kitties, kitties," she intoned. Rhonda's eyes filled and she leaned toward her. "Why honey, what would we ever do with those kitties?"

At that point, Kate rose and suggested they take Rhonda down to the cafeteria for coffee. I said I would stay with Carol for awhile, and all those sad and faithful women filed out. I took Rhonda's chair. Carol fell back into that impenetrable slumber, and I watched her breathing and looked around the room and out through her window. June was giving way to July. I thought of Ted, dead three weeks now, and remembered Yolanda, gone since November. There were still three more patients I needed to visit in their homes that afternoon. I took Carol's puffy hand in mine and held it. "Carol, I have to go now. I will come back again." I laid her hand across her chest and touched her cheek. At the door I stopped, turned toward the rustling of sheets. One last time those hazel eyes held me. "I love you, I love you, I love you…"

She died on a Friday. After work, entangled in rush hour traffic on my way to collect my youngest daughter, Moira, from her Irish babysitter, I could not bear the drone of public radio. Heading west, the setting sun in my eyes, I popped in a tape. Chris Williamson, the feminist folksinger, sang, *"Don't lose heart."*

The clouds grew more brilliant in their setting-sun purple hue and I replayed the song over and over, inching toward Moira. How to bracket that immense sorrow and be a mother to three children, a wife on a Friday night? *Shit, Carol you promised; you said we'd collaborate. And besides, I never answered the question. I don't know the answer about giving up.*

ONCE AGAIN, JANE, the oncology chaplain, and I sat side by side in a wooden pew. Carol's memorial service took place in a little white church at the end of the block on which I had lived till I was 16. The garden adjoining the church had been a mecca to us as kids; it was the place where my friends and I had brought some of the first Barbie dolls ever manufactured by Mattel and staged elaborate plots among the flowers. The fact that it was a Protestant church and we Catholic kids had no right to trespass made it all the more delicious. But we never dared to penetrate the inner sanctum.

Members of the Lesbian Health Alliance were scattered throughout the small chapel. They offered stories and filled in the blanks about what had happened after Carol abandoned Dr. Patel and orthodox treatment. Testimonies to her bravery and humor abounded. And many stood and eulogized the precancerous, vibrant, and puckish Carol. An old friend from Iowa, a gentle guy whose voice kept breaking, shared something about a frozen fish shipped from Alaska that somehow thawed en route to its destination. By the roar that went up from the congregation, it was clear it was a well-worn and much-loved tale.

The same man and childhood friend of Carol's finished with a burning reading of Millay's poem, "Dirge Without Music."

We were invited back to their home to continue the celebration of her life. I could not go; I had patients waiting. To conclude the service, Johnny Mathis sang "Unforgettable." I put my arm through Jane's and held tightly. As we left, I stopped to pick up one of the memorial cards on the table. To the left there was a poster-sized reproduction of a black-and-white photo: Carol at her doctoral graduation, pre-diagnosis and treatment. Carol with a full head of honey-blond hair, head tilted back, laughing in a black cocktail dress and stiletto heels. Great legs. After 15 years, unforgettable—in every way.

Susie's Story

~

Linda L. Lindeke, *PhD, RN, CNP*

Susie had a degenerative metabolic storage disease and lived on a farm quite far from the urban medical center. I knew her for 20 years.

As a pediatric nurse practitioner, I helped coordinate Susie's care and support her family. I didn't do anything special in caring for Susie except to help them at various points in time when they needed a listening ear, or an advocate. Sometimes I'd explain to staff at Susie's school about her condition or therapies. Occasionally I communicated with social workers and physicians, and helped the family negotiate various systems for services. I was always so impressed with how this family kept Susie as part of everyday life despite her nonverbal and progressively dependent state. They kept her at home, with only very occasional respite for family vacations. I tried to support the family in maintaining their routines and priorities while they coped with Susie's degenerative disease.

One Saturday morning a couple of years ago, I received a phone call from her dad that Susie had died that morning. She was 23 years old. At last, she was no longer suffering from this dreadful disease.

That morning we talked a long time about what Susie was like when I first met her as a happy, active, blond three-year-old little girl. We recalled how difficult—almost impossible—it had been to find out her diagnosis and look ahead to her future of progressive debilitation. But somehow this family coped and raised her brother and sister, who are now in their twenties and doing very well. We talked about the many years Susie had at home with her family, going to school on a school bus and enjoying life in whatever way was possible given her circumstances.

I was honored to be someone who could share this most private and poignant moment in Susie's life—and death—by having this connection over so many years with them and with their special little girl. Knowing Susie and her family has made a difference in how I work with other children and families. I told her parents I would continue to talk about her with my students. My main intervention with this family was being there from year to year to listen and to tell them what wonderful parents they were. This was a very remarkable family…and the world has many remarkable families that we as nurses are privileged to know and work with.

The Longest Watch

~

Bonnie Jarvis-Lowe, RN

LITTLE DID I know that Christmas Day 1998 would be my most memorable Christmas—all because of Norman, an elderly gentleman on our palliative care unit.

Norman was a proud man. He was a veteran of the Second World War. He had been a farmer all his life, raising five sons and four daughters. And he was a widower, but most of his family lived within driving distance. He could no longer care for himself and could not keep his pain medication straight.

This Christmas was going to be his last and he knew it, as did his family.

After our morning report, all of us nurses made our rounds, dispensed medication, soaked up our patients' compliments, had pictures taken with them, admired their gifts, and generally overdosed on goodies and chocolates.

They were a wonderful group of patients that Christmas. We prepared the medications for each patient who was leaving on a day pass, including Norman. He said his family was coming, so his caregivers got him dressed in his Legion blazer and gray flannel dress pants, with his beret nicely perched on his shock of white hair. Such a quiet man: shy in a way, but so loving, caring, courteous, and kind to all he knew.

One by one the families came to sign the out-on-pass slip; one by one the patients left, bundled up against the chill of the day. They would be back by eight PM, they assured us.

Those who were too ill to go home for the day received all kinds of special attention from visiting family and nurses. A young man who walked with his IV pole and was fighting for his life had a half-dozen young women in attendance, all healthy-looking friends who came to help their classmate get through a rough day.

As I settled down to do the day's mundane paperwork, I noticed one of my senior team members coming toward me, flustered and near tears.

"Nobody has come for Norman," she said. "Where are they all?"

She went on to tell me he was parked in his wheelchair in his special place—a strategic spot from where he could see the elevator doors and the stairway entrance. He wouldn't leave his parking spot. But nobody came.

By 11 AM, it was time for Plan B. We manned the phones and tried to locate somebody for Norman. Nobody answered the calls. Norman refused to eat.

He was having dinner at home, he said. But nobody came.

Time wore on. We jokingly asked him to come and dine with a bevy of beautiful nurses. He smiled and said, "No, they'll be here." But they weren't.

Norman took his pain medication, allowed himself to be wheeled around to visit a few patients he knew, and returned to his parking spot. Still, nobody came. Our hearts were breaking for this dear old man. By mid-afternoon, Norman's head was drooping. We knew he had to be hungry. What could we do? So the phone calls started again. Still, nobody answered.

The young man, with his friends in tow, gave Norman several little wrapped Christmas gifts, bought him a cold drink, and made conversation with him. Norman would not break his vigil, though. He would wait. He knew the roads were clear; he knew the usual time his family had Christmas dinner; but he would not give up. Still, nobody came.

Soon the twilight of the winter evening descended on our little hospital, making the Christmas lights twinkle and reflect off the snow on the windowsills and patio. Cars began to return with our patients. The air was quiet as people were put to bed telling us stories of their wonderful day.

The time came when, as team leader, I had to talk to Norman. He had to get out of that chair. He was exhausted.

With a crew of supportive nurses around me, I coaxed him to come to his room and open the gifts that had piled up on his bed throughout the day. He reluctantly let us take him there. We had punch and cake, and encouraged him to open his gifts. We brought other patients in to enjoy it all with him. We took his picture.

Norman was tired and heartbroken. Half of us were in tears, and when he started to cry, soon we all were in tears.

Before I left the hospital that evening, I went to say good night to Norman. During our talk, I asked him what his job had been when he was in the service during the Second World War.

"I was a gunner and a lookout, mostly," he said, his eyes brimming with tears. "But you know, nurse, this was the longest watch I ever did."

Norman passed away four days after Christmas, quietly, in the middle of the night. In his hand was one of the little gift boxes the young man had given to him on Christmas Day.

Acknowledgment of Permissions

"It Doesn't Have to Hurt," by Susan Riker Dolan and Audrey iker Vizzard, is reprinted with the kind permission of Kaplan Publishing. The story is adapted from *The End-of-Life Advisor: Personal, Legal, and Medical Considerations for a Peaceful, Dignified Death.*

Reader's Guide

1. In "The First Patient," Anne Webster relates the story of her first encounter as a nurse with death. If you're a nurse, describe some of the fears and hopes you experienced when you first cared for a dying patient. Can you relate to the student experience of this nurse in terms of the sense of responsibility and feelings of inadequacy in caring for dying patients? Have you perceived differences in the ways that nurses and physicians cope with dying patients? Can physicians also have feelings of guilt, remorse, inadequacy and failure? What are some of the ways in which experienced nurses care for dying patients as opposed to how novice nurses provide such care? What are some of the most important lessons for novice nurses?

2. As related in "Mel's Story," healing opportunities occur for patients and families as nurses encourage them to "tell their story" and acknowledge their feelings. Why is it important to give patients and families the opportunity to tell their story? When is it appropriate for a nurse or another person to share her or his own stories?

3. In Adrienne Zurub's "Tender Mercy," we learn the death of a patient may exacerbate feelings of loss related to the death of a nurse's own family member. If you are a nurse, how have you reconciled the death of a patient when it reawakens your own personal loss? Have you ever felt that other members of the health care team are unaware of your personal emotional pain? How best can colleagues offer support in this situation? In this story, do you believe the nurse expresses normal grief or complicated grief following the death of her mother?

4. Consider the story "A Nurse's Recovery from Grief" and how author Keith Carlson dealt with loss. Grieving is a process with physical emotional, psychological and spiritual manifestations. What manifestations of grief have you experienced in the death of loved ones and patients? What do you understand about grief based on your own experiences? What has helped you to deal with your grief? How can nurses support each other in the grief process? Have you found any benefit to having loved and lost someone dear to you?

5. Consider Cortney Davis's story "House Call." What aspects of house calls/home visits are most difficult for nurses? What aspects of house calls/home visits are most rewarding? What do nurses learn about the patient and their families by visiting the home and

how does this inform nursing care? How can nurses support children in their experience of death and what implications will this possibly have in their perspectives regarding dying and death?

6. In "There Are No Coincidences," think about how trust was created between Patrice Piretti and her patient. The level of caring between patient and nurse can influence their individual journeys and demonstrate respect for each others' human spirit. This mutual respect creates an environment of trust which strengthens the relationship and contributes to the healing process for both. What creates a close bond between patients and nurses? Who benefits from this bond? How do nurses use their intuitive knowledge in the care of a patient? How does this knowledge more fully inform nurses about the needs of their patients? How do you create heart to heart connections with people? What does this connection feel like when it happens? Do you think that "there are no coincidences" in life, that everything does happen for a reason? Are some people brought into our lives to help us grow emotionally and spiritually?

7. Bette served as a great inspiration in the story "She Inspired Me" through her positive attitude and upbeat demeanor. What have you learned about dying with dignity from your patients? How can nurses promote a death with dignity? How has patient's appreciation

for your care influenced your caregiving ability or affected feelings of professional burnout? Has caring for a dying patient, as portrayed in this story, influenced your philosophy of life? What are some of the most important lessons you have learned from someone who is dying?

8. In "Never Too Late" and "An End to the Madness," the issue of a DNR order is raised. What are some of the challenges when dealing with a patient who does or does not wish to be cared for with "extreme measures" or with a patient who does or does not have a DNR? How do you deal with friends or families whose wishes contradict the patient's own end-of-life care instructions?

About the Editor

DEBORAH WITT SHERMAN, PhD, APRN, ANP-BC, ACHPN, FAAN, is Professor and Assistant Dean of Research, Faculty for the Developing Center of Excellence in Palliative Care Research at University of Maryland's School of Nursing. She was previously an associate professor with tenure in the College of Nursing at New York University where she coordinated the first nurse practitioner palliative care master's program in the United States. Dr. Sherman's background in critical care nursing, hospice nursing, and her certifications as an adult and palliative care nurse practitioner, as well as her research focus on populations with life threatening illness, are foundational to her expertise and commitment to palliative care. Dr. Sherman is coauthor of the award-winning textbook, *Palliative Care Nursing: Quality Care to the End of Life.*

About the Contributors

LISA AFFATATO, RN, obtained her degree from Farmingdale College and is pursuing a master's degree from Stony Brook University. She is currently employed at Huntington Hospital as a staff/charge nurse on a med/surg floor, and she is certified in medical/surgical nursing. Affatato was the first staff RN to be appointed as chairperson for the Council of Nursing Honors at Huntington Hospital. In addition, she has served as chairperson for Community Outreach for the Academy of Medical/Surgical Nursing. Affatato was nominated in 2007 for the Magnet Nurse Award at Huntington Hospital. She speaks at many high school career days and serves as preceptor for new graduates and nursing students.

SARAH BURNS, RN, graduated from Northern Michigan University's Nursing Program in 1985. Since then she has worked at hospitals in Massachusetts, Michigan, and Texas. Currently she works in a medical intensive care unit at The University of Michigan Hospital.

KEITH CARLSON, RN, is a nurse, consultant, writer, and blogger who lives in New England. His work as a nurse has centered on ambulatory care, care management, chronic illness, and hospice. His widely read blog, Digital Doorway, can be found at http://digitaldoorway.blogspot.com.

PATRICIA COATES KAVANAUGH, RN, has spent more than three decades as a nurse, including 37 years at the University of Illinois Hospital and many years as a home healthcare field nurse.

PATO COG, RN, received an associate's degree in nursing from Prairie State College; a bachelor of science degree from College of St. Francis (now University of St. Francis); and sat for the original Hospice Certification (CHRN). Previously, Pato worked in commercial art and accounting. As a hospice nurse, Pato has found purpose: to give so that others feel healed.

LUCY MAY J. COLEGADO, RN, earned her BSN degree from Adventist University of the Philippines in 1993. She has been a bedside nurse for more than ten years. The first four years of her career were spent working in a private hospital in Pasay City, Philippines, in labor and delivery, pediatrics, and ICU. She has been working in a Southern California medical center for the past six years, the first few months in a medical surgical ICU and then in a medical intermediate telemetry unit.

PATRICK COLWELL, RN, former computer systems guy, fulfilled a lifelong dream when he changed careers into nursing. He is the author of *Mystic Nurse*, which describes his years working in emergency nursing.

CORTNEY DAVIS, RN, is a nurse practitioner in women's health. She is the author of *I Knew a Woman* (Random House), which won the Center for the Book's 2002 award for non-fiction. Co-editor of two anthologies of poetry and prose by nurses, *Between the Heartbeats* and *Intensive Care* (University of Iowa Press), Davis has been awarded an NEA Poetry Fellowship and two Connecticut Commission Poetry Grants. "First Night" will also appear in "The Heart's Truth: Essays on the Art of Nursing" (Kent State University Press, 2009).

MARY DELISLE-BERRY, RN, has been a nurse for more than 25 years. She is currently part of the neuro/oncology team at the University of Michigan. Her experience in nursing includes bedside hospital nursing on acute medical and surgical units, ICU, and neuro rehab. She has managed a sub-acute treatment facility for brain injured patients, supervised a cardiac ICU, and spent nine years as a case manager for hospice.

GERALDINE GORMAN, RN, PhD, is an assistant professor in the College of Nursing at the University of Illinois at Chicago. She holds a doctorate in nursing and a master's degree in English literature. She also practices as hospice nurse, and is interested in the application of shiatsu for end-of-life care.

KATHY INGALLINERA, RN, graduated from the Medical College of Virginia School of Nursing in 1983 with a BSN. After working a year in Connecticut, she returned to MCV as an RN in the medical-respiratory ICU, spending twelve years at the bedside. Receiving her MSN in primary care in 1996, she moved to Sitka, Alaska, where she works as a family nurse practitioner.

KAREN KLEIN, RN, obtained her BSN from Adelphi University, graduating magna cum laude. Her varied nursing experience over the past 24 years includes ER/trauma, pediatrics, interventional radiology, telemetry, ICU, home infusion and occupational health. She is a certified emergency nurse, an AHA CPR/First Aid Instructor and has been published by *Nursing Spectrum* magazine.

KAREN KUPSCO, CHPN, is an off-shift patient care manager for Rainbow Hospice in Park Ridge, Illinois. Having served in various capacities in the hospice field (including case manager, team manager and marketing representative), she plans to attain nurse practitioner certification in the specialties of adult and palliative care.

BONNIE LOWE-JARVIS, RN, is a trained nurse, graduating from the Grace General Hospital School of Nursing in 1969. Now retired, she spent most of her thirty-year nursing career in Nova Scotia. She began her career in nursing in the operating room and then switched to bedside nursing after seventeen years.

EMILY J. MCGEE, RN, MSN, APRN-BC, NREMT-P, is a flight nurse at Aero Med in Grand Rapids, Michigan. She is also a nurse and captain in the U.S. Army Reserves, and works as an emergency room nurse practitioner. In her spare time, Emily writes about flight nursing at www.crzegrl.net. Her hobbies include anything involving massive amounts of adrenaline.

CARA MUHLHAHN, CNM, is a graduate of Columbia University School of Nursing, and SUNY Downstate Health Science Center in Brooklyn's Midwifery Education Program. She has practiced as a midwife since obtaining her Certificate of Nurse-Midwifery in 1991. Prior to starting her private practice in 1996, Cara practiced midwifery at Beth Israel Medical Center, and at Maternity Center, Inc., Manhattan's Birthing Center, both in New York, New York. "God Bless the Child" is adapted from the forthcoming *Labor of Love: A Midwife's Memoir.*

MADELEINE MYSKO, RN, is a graduate of The Writing Seminars of The Johns Hopkins University, where she now teaches creative writing. Her work has appeared in *The Hudson Review, Shenandoah, Bellevue Literary Review, The Baltimore Sun, American Journal of Nursing,* and elsewhere. Her novel *Bringing Vincent Home* (Plain

View Press) is based on her experiences as an Army nurse on the burn ward during the Vietnam War.

NKIRU ONYENWE OKAMMOR, BSN, was born in Brooklyn, New York, and spent her childhood in Nigeria. She earned associate's degrees in nursing and in science from CUNY Medgar Evers College and a BSN from SUNY Downstate Medical Center. She currently is working on a graduate nursing course at University of Michigan (UOM). Okammor started her nursing career in 2003 and currently works at University of Michigan's hospital in internal medicine. She is an advocate for nursing education, quality, and patient safety.

PATRICE PIRETTI, RN-C, BSN, MPA, graduated from C.W. Post Campus of Long Island University with a BS and MPA in Health Care Administration. She earned a BSN in nursing from Molloy College. She began her nursing career in a local community hospital and soon became aware that she wanted to become a public health nurse. She worked for the Suffolk County Department of Health and Huntington Hospital's Dolan Family Health Center. During this time, she achieved certification in ambulatory care nursing. She currently works as an evening supervisor for Huntington Hospital.

ANGELA POSEY-ARNOLD, RN, is an award-winning published Christian author and retired RN. Angela has been widely published, including two books, many short stories, articles, devotionals and poetry. Her work is featured in *Faithwriters* and *Guidepost's Angels on Earth* magazines. Angela is also a contributing writer for the popular e-mag www.4Him2U.com. Her latest book is *The Nightingale Protocol.* Visit her website www. angelaposeyarnold.com.

TERRY RATNER, RN, MFA, is a registered nurse, freelance writer, and educator in Phoenix, Arizona. She teaches creative writing in a variety of settings, from community colleges to a school for the homeless, to wellness communities. She has published numerous personal essays, cover stories, interviews, and book reviews for both national and local publications. Her current work in progress, a series of fifteen essays introduced with black and white photos, deals with issues of family and identity. She is editor of *Reflections on Doctors: Nurses' Stories about Physicians and Surgeons.* www.terryratner.com

SUSAN RIKER DOLAN, JD, RN, CHA, is a registered nurse and an attorney. Susan practiced healthcare and corporate law and is licensed as an attorney and nurse in Indiana, Illinois, and Wisconsin. She served as executive director for a national hospice organization, is a healthcare consultant and a broadcast host for satellite radio station ReachMD XM 157, the channel for medical professionals. Susan is co-author of *The End-of-Life Advisor: Personal, Legal, and Medical Considerations for a Peaceful, Dignified Death.*

RACHEL SHINABARGER, RN, has been a nurse for about 15 years. She attended Bryan Memorial Hospital School of Nursing in Lincoln, Nebraska. She now works on the surgical floor at Kadlec Hospital in Richland, Washington, where she's been here for almost 10 years. Shinabarger began her career on medical-telemetry floors, but found a home among surgical patients. Her greatest love is teaching patients, families, and nurses. She teaches a pre-op total hip and knee class for planned surgeries and also regularly precepts new nurses coming to the floor.

IRMA VELASQUEZ-KRESSNER, RNC, is passionate about her nursing career, which she began after emigrating from South America. She is currently pursuing her BSN/MSN at Thomas Edison State College.

AUDREY RIKER VIZZARD, RN, EdD, is a nurse and clinical psychologist. She is a former adjunct professor of psychology at Purdue University and the author of many books and articles. She served as a hospice volunteer and facilitates an ongoing Good Grief Group for seniors actively dealing with caregiving and loss. Audrey also serves as the director of her family foundation. Audrey is co-author of *The End-of-Life Advisor: Personal, Legal, and Medical Considerations for a Peaceful, Dignified Death.*

ANNE WEBSTER, RN, has held positions in Critical Care and Nursing Administration during the past twenty-five years. Her work has recently appeared in *The Poetry of*

Nursing: Commentaries and Poems of Leading Nurse Poets and *Rattle. A History of Nursing,* her poetry collection, is forthcoming from Kennesaw State University Press.

ADRIENNE ZURUB, RN, MA, CNOR, is a speaker, comedian, actor, and poet. She is the author of the memoir Notes from the *Mothership: The Naked Invisibles.* She served on the Cleveland Clinic open-heart team for more than twenty years. Her blog can be found at http://adriennezurub.typepad.com.